IGOR KLEKH

ADVENTURES IN THE SLAVIC KITCHEN
– A BOOK OF ESSAYS WITH RECIPES –

GLAGOSLAV PUBLICATIONS

ADVENTURES IN THE SLAVIC KITCHEN:
A BOOK OF ESSAYS WITH RECIPES

by Igor Klekh

Translated from Russian
by Slava I. Yastremski and Michael M. Naydan

© 2016, Igor Klekh

© 2016, Glagoslav Publications, United Kingdom

Glagoslav Publications Ltd
88-90 Hatton Garden
EC1N 8PN London
United Kingdom

www.glagoslav.com

ISBN: 978-1-78437-996-4

A catalogue record for this book is available
from the British Library.

This book is in copyright. No part of this publication may be reproduced, stored in a retrieval system or transmitted in any form or by any means without the prior permission in writing of the publisher, nor be otherwise circulated in any form of binding or cover other than that in which it is published without a similar condition, including this condition, being imposed on the subsequent purchaser.

IGOR KLEKH

ADVENTURES IN THE SLAVIC KITCHEN

– A BOOK OF ESSAYS WITH RECIPES –

TRANSLATED BY SLAVA I. YASTREMSKI AND MICHAEL M. NAYDAN

*This book is dedicated to the memory
of Slava Yastremski (1952-2015),
a wonderful colleague, great friend,
and beautiful human being.*

Acknowledgements

First of all the translators want to thank the author, Igor Klekh, who not only has written so eloquently about Slavic foods but also frequently has treated us with sumptuous samples of Russian and Ukrainian dishes to support the points he wants to make in his book from a practical perspective.

The translators also want to thank their wives for their constant support during the long process of preparing this book for publication.

Introduction

AN ADVENTURE IN
THE SLAVIC KITCHEN WITH IGOR KLEKH

Igor Klekh is an accomplished Russian writer, the author of seven books of prose, essays, and criticism. Since 1994 Klekh has resided in Moscow, but as a writer he was formed in the western Ukrainian city of Lviv, which, as a result of its proximity to Poland and the rest of Europe, has always had freer contacts with the West, even during the Soviet period. Historically many cultural traditions have been intersecting and interrelating in Galicia and Transcarpathia, mutually enriching each other in striking ways. As a writer Klekh was influenced by both the great Russian literary tradition and the languages and dialects of East-Central Europe. Being a phenomenon of the multicultural environment of Galician Ukraine, Klekh to a certain degree represents at least in part that phenomenon of marginalized colonial writing when the literary culture of the colonized parts of the empire, with its unique perspectives, seemingly overtakes and influences the center. From the cultural perspective the region can be seen as a proverbial melting pot, in which Igor Klekh cooks his multicultural dishes and offers his meditations on the significance of various dishes in Slavic national cultures, particularly Russian and Ukrainian.

The book comprises a cultural study of the role food plays in the formation and expression of a nation's character. It focuses primarily on Russian and Ukrainian kitchens but discusses them in the context of international food practices. Some of the essays have appeared previously in various Russian periodicals as well as in other of Klekh's publications and were later included in the bestselling *The Book of Food* (published in 2007) to round out his cultural discourse on Slavic foods. In our translation the book is divided into four parts: "The Philosophy of the Kitchen," which discusses the significance of food in national cultures; "Cultural Dictionary of East Slavic Food," which discusses foods that are quintessential for the Ukrainian and Russian food cultures (such as *salo* [pig lard] and *bliny* [thin crepe-like pancakes]) as well as the consumption of alcohol and hangover recipes; "Seasonal Culinary Art," which is dedicated to seasonal dishes, such as winter soups—borsht and *shchi* and Siberian *pelmeni*, summer salads, autumn pickled and marinated vegetables, etc.; and "Cities and Dishes," essays based on Klekh's travels to different European and Near Eastern countries as a writer for *Geo Magazine*.

Klekh's book is not a traditional recipe cookbook, although it offers recipes for all the major dishes in the kitchens of the Eastern Slavs. It is rather a collection of essays on the cultural implications of particular dishes and foods, such as borsht, pig lard, mushrooms, etc. Most of the essays that comprise the book are written in the genre of the informal aphoristic literary essay, which started with Bacon, who described the genre as "grains of salt which will rather give an appetite than offend with satiety." In his essays Klekh continues the rich essayistic tradition of twentieth-century Western and Russian writers and thinkers, such as Kafka, Joyce, Virginia Woolf, and Nabokov, and perhaps most of all Borges, who has had the greatest influence on Klekh as well as on his entire generation. Similarly to Borges, Klekh's essays blur the boundaries between genres and styles. Most of Klekh's essays in the section "Cultural Dictionary of East Slavic Food" are about one particular food taken in its totality: in all the complexity of the word's semantic meanings, its phonetic sound, and the visual image the name of the food denotes. Klekh explains this seeming postmodernist paradox by the significance that food and its preparation play in the cultural formation of all nations: "The kitchen is one of the most ancient performance theaters, especially in the case of fundamental dishes prepared with a minimum of means: flour, water, fire" ("The Origins of the Kitchen"), which is best illustrated by the essay called "Blin." If we accept flour as a kind of dust and a product of the earth, the preparation of these crepe-like pancakes will include three of the four primary elements, which comprise the basis of life. The very process of making *bliny* becomes for Klekh a cosmological myth of creation. The typical Russian dish is transformed into a mythic primary element of Russian culture. Klekh begins his essay with a visual image of the pancake: "If you project the cross-section of the world tree onto the Russian kitchen… you'll get a *blin*" ("The Blin"). Thus, a *blin* becomes the axis mundi of the Russian cultural landscape. Klekh presents his philosophical musings on the more profound nature of Slavic foods in a wonderful style and thereby offers fascinating insights into Russian and Ukrainian cultures.

Even when he provides a recipe, Klekh creates a cultural-historical narrative about the origin and significance of that particular dish for the people of a certain country. For example, in discussing borsht, he writes: "There is something pan-Slavic in this dish. Borsht is a metaphor for summer, for which every Slav waits and longs. That is why borsht has to be served not just hot, but scorching hot, scorching with the afternoon summer heat" ("Formula for Borsht"). Admitting that borsht was appropriated by other cultures (Soviet Russian, before all the rest), Klekh returns to the genuine Ukrainian formula that requires the achievement of an appropriate degree of spiciness, red and black peppers, cloves, and crushed garlic ground with sea salt and Ukrainian *salo*. Klekh takes the reader on a fascinating culinary adventure full of exotic names such as *khmeli-suneli, pechenya, vereshchaka, zavyvanets, verguny, imam-bayaldy, okroshka*, etc., and accomplishes daring culinary border-crossings such as the Russian appropriation of the French salad Oliver or the relationship between Ukrainian *vareniki* (cottage cheese or cherry dumplings) and their Turkish prototype.

In his book Klekh focuses on foods and dishes of primarily two Slavic peoples: the Russians and Ukrainians, but he also shows the influences, borrowings, and modifications that each nation has made to the kitchens of its neighbors as well as interactions with other kitchens of the world: the French, Chinese, Italian, American (mostly in its fast-food manifestation), and others. While standing at the stove stirring the ingredients in his large cultural pot of Russian-Ukrainian borsht or sprinkling various vegetable dishes with multi-cultural spices, Klekh shares with his readers his thoughts on the significance this or that dish has in one of the Slavic cultures.

Klekh writes his book not only from within the culinary traditions of the Eastern Slavic peoples. His book is also steeped in the cooking and food consumption practices that were developed during seventy-four years of the Soviet regime and have continued to dominate Russian and Ukrainian food cultures even today. One can say that nowadays we, to my personal surprise, can witness a strong nostalgia for the simple foods of the Soviet times, such as we find in Klekh's book – "marine-style macaroni" or "sardines in tomato sauce." This nostalgia is a yearning for lost and idealized childhood, and in his book Klekh pays tribute to it, wistfully discussing mothers' cooking, the taste of homemade jams and pies, pickled mushrooms and hot winter soups. Some aspects of these cooking cultures may be confusing for the English-speaking audience. For example, both Russian and Ukrainian cultures until recently have been focused determinately on home-cooking with their own versions of Betty Crocker and Julia Child kinds of cooking gurus – William Pokhlebkin and Elena Molokhovets, for example. During Soviet times people mostly stayed away from going out to eat. Restaurants were expensive, and people would go to them only on special occasions. We should also remember that the average family's budget did not allow for frequent meals outside the home, and "child-friendly" restaurants were almost non-existent. The food offered by the public cafeterias and low-end restaurants, to which Klekh refers as *obshchepit* (Public Food Production and Supply System), was, as a rule, of very low quality, and even those were quite sparse. As the popular joke went: "Someone asks how was the food at lunch at a public cafeteria, and another answers: 'First of all it tasted like shit, and secondly there was too little of it.'" Lunches were taken out at the workers' cafeterias or buffets, in which the food was no better, but at least it was cheap. In addition to that, with almost non-existent nutrition and food safety control, people had serious reservations about eating out. The majority firmly believed that they could prepare tastier and healthier food at home, although home cooking was complicated by the limited assortment of products in grocery stores and the high prices for better quality food at the farmers' markets. With the exception of bread and milk, which were purchased fresh every day, the ingredients were bought once a week and the dishes were prepared for several days in advance, using all parts of the purchased products. This historical fact is also reflected in the book. On several occasions Klekh discusses the fact that bones can be used for soups while the meat is used for pie filling; or while you fry the body of the fish, its head can be used for making soup. Surprisingly this practice that grew out of necessity in Soviet Russia now attracts the attention of environmentally conscious food theorists and practitioners who see it as a way of finding sustainability in the food preparation process in today's world, which can help to eliminate the danger of depleting the world food resources.

No cultural study of food consumption in Russia (and other Eastern Slavic countries, as a matter of fact) can avoid a discussion of the use (or abuse) of alcohol, and Klekh is no exception. In the aphoristic essay "Vodka as Pure Alcohol" he states that "In Russia to drink is a matter of honor, conscience, and reason… Vodka – also called *horilka* (burner), *gor'kaia* (bitter), *palenka* (fire-water), by its appearance is indistinguishable from water (and, after all, you must drink water, pure as a tear, but 40° proof!)." The excessive drinking results in a hangover, and Klekh examines this phenomenon in "The Metaphysics of a Hangover" and offers necessary remedies in "Hangover Cookery."

Another important factor in food preparation that Klekh discusses in his book is "seasonal culinary," that is, the use of vegetables and fruits according to their peak seasons to get most out of them in terms of vitamins and nutrients. His reflections on "seasonal culinary art" can be seen as one of Klekh's original contributions to the discussion of the art of cooking. During Soviet times "seasonal culinary art" was an inevitable necessity – people had to rely on the meager supply of fresh produce available in grocery stores. In winter and spring months it was almost impossible to find any fresh fruit or tomatoes or cucumbers. People could try the farmers markets, to where these products were brought from Georgia or Azerbaijan or, more rarely, from Central Asia, but the prices were extraordinarily high. As a result, in the winter months consumers' choice for the most part was limited to cabbage, potatoes, and onions. All over the Soviet Union, as much as possible, people grew fruit and vegetables on their own. I encountered this practice in 1999 when I was teaching as a Fulbright scholar at the University of Tver, a historic city halfway between Moscow and St. Petersburg. My hosts, full professors at that university, received a "hefty" salary equivalent to $40 and $30 a month respectively (they were a married couple and she received $10 less for being a woman. So much for gender equality in the former workers' paradise!) The couple lived in a village two commuter train stops from the city and grew all their vegetables, spices, and some fruit (strawberries, raspberries, etc.) on their tiny private plot. They made jams, pickled cabbage and mushrooms, and dried spices for winter. If people did not have summer or private land lots, which they could cultivate, they bought fruit and vegetables in extra quantities at the local markets in the summer and early fall when the prices were much lower, so they could prepare and store them for the winter. That is why Klekh's book offers recipes for all kinds of jams and preserves, pickled and marinated cucumbers, mushrooms, cabbage, "eggplant caviar," home-made liqueurs, etc.

 For Klekh the main distinction of the Slavic kitchens is their "sour" or "pickled" character, that is, the prevalence of "sour" dishes, such as Russian *shchi* (pickled cabbage soup), Ukrainian borsht with the use of tomato paste, Polish *bigos* (a stewed cabbage dish with all kinds of meats and spices). The "sourness" of the Slavic kitchens presented certain cultural problems in translation. In Russian we have "sour" or "salted" cabbage, which is not the same as the sauerkraut that you can find in American supermarkets. The same goes for cucumbers, which in Russian can be "salted" or "semi-salted," and Klekh draws a clear difference between "salted" and marinated mushrooms, which are nowadays sold in the stores. We decided to go with "pickled" as the closest equivalent for cabbage, cucumbers, and mushrooms.

Another important thing that should be pointed out about Russian and Ukrainian cooking cultures is that they are meat-oriented, with Russians using beef and Ukrainians – pork as their main meats. At the same time vegetables such as cabbage for the Russians and beets for the Ukrainians play an important, if not crucial, role in their national cuisines, because they are used as the main ingredients for what you might call a national soup – cabbage for the Russian *shchi* and beets for the Ukrainian borsht.

It is also worth mentioning that Slavic people have a very different concept of "healthy food" if we compare it to American cooking culture. I must say that the Slavs are right in saying that nowadays their food is, generally speaking, better tasting and healthier than what is imported from the West because they do not use artificial ingredients often found in Western food products. On the other hand, the claims that *salo* (pig lard) or vodka can actually fight bad cholesterol may seem far-fetched for an American reader. But why not be adventurous and try?

Let's consider one of the most popular and widely used ingredient in Slavic cooking cultures, which usually puts fear in the hearts of American food consumers – wild mushrooms. Russians, Ukrainians, Poles, and Lithuanians fry mushrooms, add them to soups and salads, pickle and marinate them (and in these last two forms mushrooms are considered to be the best chaser after a drink, especially a shot of vodka, for example). Russians or Ukrainians either pick the mushrooms in the woods or buy them at farmers' markets. In the late summer and early fall thousands of people hike through forests to gather mushrooms. Most know which ones are safe to eat or to pickle, where the woods can be environmentally unsafe, and what time of the year and day are the best for mushroom picking. The Slavic people have a definite mushroom hierarchy with so-called "white mushrooms" (Boletus mushrooms also known as penny bun, porcino, or cep) occupying the top spot. In fact when a Slavic person says "mushroom," he or she most likely means a Boletus; the "white mushrooms" sold in American supermarkets are not even considered to be real mushrooms at all because they have no taste. Poles and Lithuanians call Boletus the king of mushrooms. The Boletus mushrooms are best for frying and soup making. The honey fungus and "little fox" (a type of chanterelle) mushrooms are considered the best for pickling. Mushroom dishes could be of a great interest for vegetarians, but where would you find Boletus mushrooms in America?

Not only the consumption of certain products in Slavic food culture appear exotic and unusual to the Western reader (something on the level with the popular TV show Bizzare Foods with Andrew Zimmern on the Travel Channel) but also certain names of Slavic foods need to be explained, for example such word as "kielbasa" (pronounced "kolbasa" in Russian and "kovbasa" in Ukrainian). While in English kielbasa means a particular type of East European sausage (such as Polish kielbasa), in Russian it stands for a generic word for all types of sausages. All Russian kielbasas are divided into two basic types: so-called "boiled sausages" that include Bologna-type sausages, with "Doctor's" and "Choice" sausages being the most popular, and hard hot- and cold-smoked sausages (as the type of Italian hard salami or chorizo). Or the word "kasha," which in addition to the universally accepted term for buckwheat groats, also is a generic term for all types of cereals, porridges, and groats. We should also remember that cold cereals were almost non-existent in the Soviet Union. In addition to buckwheat kasha, Klekh also discusses "kashitsy," the hot thin porridges, the most popular (and most hated by) among children being oat porridge. Russian and Ukrainian kitchens are quite limited in their use of spices – they mostly use just salt and pepper. Most spices used in the preparation of Russian and Ukrainian dishes come from the nations in the Caucasus Mountains, the most popular of which is *adjika* (a Georgian [referring to the former Soviet republic and now the independent country of Georgia] hot red pepper sauce)

With Russian and Ukrainian kitchens playing the central role in his book, Klekh reflects on many kitchens of other Slavic peoples who either were the part of the Soviet Union or had close political and/or cultural interactions with it. All these nations had a long and rich history of their national cooking traditions. For example, Klekh devotes a lot of attention to Polish *bigos*, Moldavian *mamalyga*, and to the use of eggplant in the kitchen of the peoples living in the Caucasus Mountains. During Soviet times Russians appropriated a lot of these dishes, making them part of the Russian holiday table. In his book Klekh restores the origin of a particular dish and discusses its significance in the national culture.

Klekh is an experienced traveler, and his encounters with national foods extend beyond the borders of the former Soviet Union and its closest neighbors. After moving from Lviv to Moscow, he worked for the travel magazine *GEO* (a kind of Russian version of *Travel and Leisure*), and for his assignments wrote about life in different countries of the world – from the former Soviet republics such as Latvia and Lithuania to Norway and Jordan. He also spent time in Germany, Switzerland, and the United States as a writer-in-residence and wrote about his experiences there. The excerpts from these essays, at least those in which he discusses dishes and foods, were included in the section "Cities and Dishes." This section serves as a fitting conclusion to this journey through Slavic kitchens and places them in the broader context of European and other world cuisines.

To maintain the linguistic flavor of the national kitchens we decided to leave the names of specific Russian and Ukrainian dishes and foods in transliteration in our translation, with a short explanation of what they are attached to them when they are used for the first time: for example, *shchi* (cabbage soup) or *halushki* (unstuffed dumplings). We also decided to use the Russian plural endings "–y" or "–i" for dishes such as *bliny* or *pelmeni*, because it seemed more natural to us than the standard English plural form with an "s," which would have turned these into awkward sounding *blins* or *pelmens*.

In light of the recent Russian-Ukrainian conflict, the translation of the book in English appears to be very timely. Klekh's work can be welcomed as a synthesis of the two traditions and as an invaluable insight into historically determined cultural interactions between the two nations. It also offers an alternative way for conflict resolution – making food, and not war. It offers an unusual look at the peaceful interaction between Russian and Ukrainian cultures and at the same time explains Russian "culinary imperialism," especially during the Soviet period. The book is expected to appeal to a diverse audience, ranging from those who are interested in cultural studies of food to those who want to try something different in their kitchen, as well as to the Russian, Ukrainian, and Polish Americans and émigré communities.

Slava I. Yastremski

PART I
The Philosophy of the Kitchen

The Origin of the Kitchen

The kitchen appeared when people first began to use fire to protect themselves against the cold and predators, and that was just as great an invention for humankind as spoken language and hand tools. In the beginning there were the hearth and stove with the tamed deity of fire; next to it a butchering table (as a kind of altar for sacrifices), and utensils. Next came the creation of a set of basic, essential food products and dishes. Finally, came the ritual of eating at the table, a repast, and feasting as a particular religious rite (that is why it was customary to thank spirits or the Creator before a meal) and the symbolism of the absence of enmity (from this fact come the "round tables" of contemporary scholars and politicians, those mass produced "clones" of the Round Table of the Knights of King Arthur). We can speak of *Homo sapiens* and the birth of civilization since the time when people began to bury other people and started to cook food (that is, they performed the revolutionary transition from the "raw" to the "cooked" in Claude Levi-Strauss' formulation[1]).

It is not surprising that the food chain formed differently in different geographic and climatic zones; even more so the differentiation of tribes living in the same zone happened because one tribe of its own volition chose to feed itself in one way, and another tribe in another: tell me what you eat, and I will tell you

---

[1] The French anthropologist Claude Levi-Strauss was one of the founders of Structuralism and famous for his studies of North American myths. His approach was based on binary oppositions that were reflected in the title of his book *The Raw and the Cooked*, 1969.

who you are. Today we witness the inverse process, but it has not changed the essence of the question: in order to cook a "global" soup you need fundamental individual "ingredients" and some firm rules. If the salt stops being salty, and a bay leaf fails to taste like a bay leaf, if you combine herring with ice cream and sprinkle it with curry, you will get nothing but swill for creatures who barely resemble people by their unique pantophagy (eating-no-matter-what-it-is), but not people as such.

Why did the astronauts in the film *Solaris*[2] tie strips of paper to a fan? Why did the Russian prince, who had grown accustomed to his life in Polovtsian captivity, suddenly come to his senses and return to rule over his people when envoys from his homeland placed a bunch of steppe sagebrush to his nose?[3] Why do not only their kitchens smell different, but the Chinese, Vietnamese, and Mongolian people themselves smell differently than the Russians with the latter's specific "cabbage-soup" Russian odor? There is no racism in this, only biochemistry and the conservatism of human nature, which biologists call imprinting, science-fiction writers – the matrix, and all the rest of people – a code. If something is intrinsic for individual people, then it must be intrinsic for entire nations. Purposeful creative activity is covertly interwoven with biochemistry and cultural memory. Food does not determine abilities, but seemingly diverts and directs them along the resultant forces of the parallelogram. That is why icon-painters observe a strict fast before painting an icon, athletes – before matches, and dancers – before performances, and why Pavarotti brings his own chef when he goes on tour. Thus, one person has a bell canto voice like no one else in the world, and another – a throaty singing voice, a third – diligence, and a fourth – inspiration, etc. In short, everything is interconnected in

---

2 A reference to the Russian film director Andrei Tarkovsky's science fiction film *Solaris*, 1972.

3 A reference to the purportedly twelfth-century folk epic *The Lay of Prince Igor's Campaign*, which became the basis for Alexander Borodin's opera *Prince Igor*, 1887/1890.

the human world as it is in the universe with the endless circulation of energy and matter.

This entire deep philosophy in shallow waters is needed just to proclaim once again: any kitchen is not just a collection of recipes, but a flexible, ramified system connected with some natural conditions and existing in unexplained relationships with all aspects of national, regional, and personal life.

That is what happens with the Russian kitchen – sometimes it overshoots, sometimes it undershoots the standards; sometimes it is sour (*kvasnoi*) patriotism[4] (which received its name from the Russian *kvas*—a bread-based brewed libation!); other times it is the sour doubt in the very existence of the Russian kitchen (borsht is Ukrainian, *pelmeni* [meat dumplings] are from China, potatoes are from America, pickled herring is from the Atlantic, etc.). And it is not a question of life on Mars! Besides nature and the population, such uncelebrated and celebrated practitioners have worked on the creation of Russian cuisine that in its best periods it has been one of the "tastiest" and most diverse kitchens in the world. The problem is that in terms of theory, only the illustrious culinary specialist and writer W.V. Pokhlebkin has articulated a systematic approach to it. It is understandable that every bird is inclined to like its own nest, therefore let's try to look at this matter from without.

In terms of the effectiveness of food, its convenience, and accessibility in the modern world, McDonald's and pizza parlors (those, figuratively speaking, unpretentious culinary Kalashnikov machine guns), or to put it differently, the almost universally established system of fast food and the use of pre-prepared food, which more and more is ready for consumption, beat everything else. In proportion to the disappearance of the peasantry with its traditional kitchen, it could not be any different from what might be expected.

---

4 "Kvasnoi" comes from the word "kvas" (a kind of Russian root beer brewed from rye bread), which is considered to be a Russian national drink. It is an ironic name for "pseudo-super patriotism" or jingoism, as an expression for all Russian, regardless how silly it can sound. "Kvasnoi" also means sour.

However, in terms of cooking, everything is different and more complex. Here the mighty culinary inertia that represents one of the most important elements of national culture continues to play an important role. Here the luminaries are the over-sophisticated and "long-playing" French and Chinese kitchens. These kitchens are Imperial, continental, totalitarian, and their hidden pathos consists of achieving maximum power over the base product – in the transformation of its taste and appearance (to feed a goose to the point it dies, to let mold eat through cheese, to bury eggs in lime for a year, to present soy as meat or fish, to decorate dishes and transform the table into some kind of theater). The "island" kitchens, that stand in opposition to them, the British and Japanese ones, are inclined to minimal interference over the taste of the original raw material (bloody roast beef, raw fish, culinary purity), although during their Imperial period, these kitchens did not shy away from violence either (the British "tenderized" pigs by pounding them while they were still alive to achieve a more palatable taste, and the Japanese acquired a taste for poisonous fish in the same way as the Chinese did for snakes). Strictly speaking, the French kitchen is the most advanced and richest variant of the so-called Mediterranean or Roman kitchen, that is, of the whole bouquet of kitchens that to some degree originated in or were influenced by the super-sophisticated kitchen of Ancient Rome. In this respect, the magnificent but less Imperial and more democratic Italian kitchen echoes and at the same time stands opposite to the French kitchen.

The Russian kitchen of the last two centuries is also an Imperial, continental kitchen that went through the school of the best French chefs after the Napoleonic invasion of 1812. Without losing its Slavic simplicity, the Russian kitchen managed in the course of two centuries to digest and appropriate so many dishes from the diet of the subjects of the Russian (and later Soviet) Empire and its near and distant neighbors (starting with borsht and *pelmeni* [Russian dumplings] and ending with shish kebab and pilaf) that it took it out of the ranks of conservative, ethnic kitchens and made it supra-national. I mean here not the expansion of exotic restaurants, which have the function strictly of entertainment all over the world (roughly speaking, they serve culinary tourism), but rather the inclusion of certain dishes for the Russian family table – their taming or *domestication.*

Every kitchen has its limitations, even taboos, as well as strong and weak points. For example, Russian wine is vodka (made of grain and not from grapes), and Russian meat is boiled or stewed beef (the Russian stove could not teach Russian women to fry meat, and you feel that to this day). However, no one can take away our vodka table with the spectacular selected hors-d'oeuvres and the rich, neutral taste of beef. Similarly, you cannot deny the huge list of soups (from cabbage soup and borsht to the Europeanized *solyanka* [vegetable and meat soup]), the richest fish and mushroom table, an entire school of pickled vegetable dishes (not the necrotic marinades) and preserves (and not pectin comfitures). The shortcoming of the latter is their excessive sweetness, but to this end we have black tea (borrowed from the Chinese and Asian Indians, and the *samovar* – from the Japanese); but it is compensated for by the freshness of garden and forest berries, by their taste, smell, and health benefits, which the foreign competitors of correctly prepared preserves do not have. Among baked goods we must point out "black" and "gray" bread (white bread also turns out well sometimes, but never as well as with Italian or French bakers), Russian *bliny* (unsweetened crepe-like thin yeast-dough pancakes), Siberian *pelmeni*, and an enormous range of meat-, fish-, vegetable-, and fruit-stuffed pies. Pastries are not our strong point. Instead we have baked kashas (especially buckwheat) and soft-boiled potatoes (sprinkled with dill and served with pickled herring or common canned stewed meat) that no one else can even try to prepare. Similarly, the Italians will never understand the Soviet "marine style" macaroni. For the contemporary Russian person, the main vegetable after cabbage and the potato is the cucumber; the main fruit is the

Antonov apple[5]; the main berry – the raspberry; the main vegetable oil – sunflower, among cultured milk products – sour cream and authentic kefir (just try to find it west of the Oder in Europe). We can go on, but the principle is clear – a filled-in space followed by a blank space as a cipher or the key to it, in a word – a menu.

Gourmets prefer to read, study, enjoy, and collect… menus! A menu is the algebra of the culinary discipline. They are collected and stored like herbaria. They are studied just as elegantly played chess games are. A culinary Sherlock Holmes can determine, studying a hundred-year-old menu, everything that took place at the dinner table that day; he can laugh at the mistakes and enjoy witticisms. In a similar way a more or less clear profile of the country, its people, the author and his times, inevitably shows through the recipes of dishes and culinary recommendations on the pages of cookbooks.

The present book does not claim to give a full picture, but simply represents an attempt to compose something like "culinary prose," which is good for reading and stirring up ideas, and with that, awakening appetite in the most literal sense of the word. It could be called "Rehabilitation of the Appetite" because, as Anton Chekhov said in his play *Ivanov*: "Humankind has thought and thought and still has not invented anything better than a pickle as a chaser for a shot of vodka."[6]

The Professor of Sour Cabbage Soup,[7] or Homage to William Pokhlebkin

Why when we think about food, which has become an obsession with us, three names inevitably rise to the surface in our native

---

5 Antonov apples are an equivalent to American Granny Smith apples.

6 Anton Chekhov's *Ivanov*, a drama in four acts, 1887. The quote is from Act 3.

7 A pejorative title applied to a person who talks about things of which he or she knows nothing. Klekh, of course, does not imply that William Pokhlebkin does not know anything about the culinary arts, he simply is playing with words here.

tradition: Gogol,[8] the drake that escapes vexed hunters[9]; the furry and flesh-eating last name Molokhvets, and Pokhlebkin, the latter a William to boot, who sat down sideways at their table? It is very simple – the table is the desk, and the sheet of paper lying before each of them turns, by magic, into a self-replenishing magic tablecloth.[10] These three are writers of different scales, destinies, and literary schools, but one common theme rises in hyperbolized form in the works of all three of them – if we say it is the theme of food and gourmet dishes, that would say nothing. A writer always represents the memory of loss, trauma, and the need to heal it. All three, as a psychoanalyst would say, wished to be fed, wished to return to the world of care and nurturing, wished to overcome the interpersonal coldness of human relations through a sense of satiety and warmth. They wrote their books because their hunger was not physiological and could not be satisfied through practical measures. They are playwrights (isn't it where the name William comes from?), while cooks, gourmets, and eaters are the directors, characters, and performers of this singular, very ancient, and constantly rewritten drama that has its origins in the mystery play. Today this drama is desacralized (and it would seem conclusively and irrevocably). Not so long ago it was customary among people to give thanks for food in a prayer, and in the Stone Age – even to ask forgiveness from the spirits of the killed animals and appease them for permission to eat their bodies. However, nowadays, the all-penetrating *obshchepit*[11]

---

8   Nikolai Gogol (1809-1852) was a Ukrainian-born Russian writer. He was most famous for his comedy *The Inspector General* and the epic satirical novel *Dead Souls*. Gogol spent twelve years in Italy, which was reflected in several of his later writings.

9   Gogol's name can be translated as "drake" (a male duck).

10 The *skatert'-samobranka* (the self-replenishing magic table cloth) is typically found in Russian folktales where the hero spreads it on a table, and, magically, all kinds of food and libations appear on it.

11 Introduced during the first Five-Year Plan, the *obshchepit* was designed to provide Soviet people with food pre-prepared at food factories and served at inexpensive public cafeterias. One of the goals of the *obshchepit* was to remove women from the kitchen so they could actively participate in the social and cultural life of the country. The food served at public cafeterias was notoriously bad.

(public food service) sweeps away the last barriers and obstacles, and this process takes place not only in life – in culinary areas of the West and the East – but also in literature and consciousness.

Fortunately, sooner or later at such moments, the mechanism of the archaic conservative counter-revolution switches on to save the values that still can be saved and to restore the connections that are being torn apart. William Pokhlebkin is one of those last Knights of the Kitchen Table. Let's remember the background – to promote female cooks to the status of Deputies of the Supreme Soviet![12] Let's remember the policy of the elimination of women homemakers as a class, a huge expansion of the Soviet system of public cafeterias, the enlargement of food production factories – huge industrial complexes and plants, and the phantasmagorical impoverishment of product variety when not just some products but even their classes and kinds disappeared without a trace, and only generic types remained: "kielbasa" (ringed sausages) in general, "meat" as such, or simply "fish." One of the possible definitions of Socialism is precisely this "impoverishment of product variety," which, in the world of food, means "nothing extra," only the necessary stuff, preferable in that it is commonly accessible. It must be said that there were some positive achievements on this path: thanks to rigid state standards, we had good bread, tolerable vodka, ice cream for everyone (thanks to the ambitious Mikoyan and his 1937 Program[13]), very decent candies and cakes, and those kinds of vegetable oil, sour cream, mustard, mayonnaise, and herring to which we have become accustomed and therefore have not needed any others. Let's forget all the cellulose ringed sausages, sour beer, deteriorated kinds of

---

12 A reference to an early revolutionary slogan attributed to Lenin, "Every female cook must learn to govern the state." Actually, Lenin was misquoted. What he said was "We know that an unskilled laborer or a cook cannot immediately get on with the job of state administration."

13 Anastas Mikoyan (1895-1978) was an old Bolshevik as well as a member of the Politburo and other high organs of the Soviet administration. In 1934 he was put in charge of the Soviet food industry and made several reforms. One of them, after a trip to the USA, was the dramatic increase in ice-cream production after he discovered that Soviet Russia lagged dramatically behind the USA in this area.

vegetables that can pass only as cattle feed, watered down milk, and it would be better left unmentioned, "schnitzel with garnish" and "Thursday is fish day" (remarkable also for the anonymity of its inventor).[14] It just happened that the 1970s turned out to be crazy about searching for something tasty, epicurean, and festive – all these were not just bought, but "obtained" – by quota, through connections, or from under the counter; and by some miracle settled, scorning all expiration dates, in the freezers of Soviet citizens. People visited each other with pleasure because it meant eating well. Restaurants with a good kitchen existed only here and there in the capitals of Soviet republics and, for some unknown reason, in unpredictable places in the provinces. The return of housewives to the kitchen had begun; husbands also started to drop in there more and more often.

Cookbooks were published every year and dutifully were bought up because, for some reason, they were considered good presents. As a rule they were distinguished by a rare obtuseness, a patchwork approach, and the mindset of their author on the level of taskmasters of the Ministry of Common Food Production. Soviet readers remember with nostalgia the late-Stalin period *Book of Tasty and Healthy Food*; it was good only for checking the spelling of outdated words and scrutinizing the color reproductions – something like a film-strip for adults about a cornucopia that was seen by discontents as a thing of the past, and by the propagandists – as a thing of the future. There were a lot of books that were similar in their simplicity and omnivorous quality to the most popular television program of that time – "The Club of Film-travelers." There were also practitioners, who supplied sometimes practical, but always clipped recipes from the "Food" columns in the woman's journals *Working Woman, Peasant Woman,* and *Health*, each of which had tens of millions of women subscribers. The recipes were more often than not cut out; they were given to be copied; homemakers exchanged

---

14 Schnitzel was a pre-prepared *obshchepit* dish, made supposedly of ground meat, but in reality contained a high percentage of bread and all kinds of other by-products.

them as children did with stamps; they were used as bookmarks in cookbooks, transforming the latter into a kind of herbarium – that is why you had to be extremely careful when taking a cookbook off the shelf, otherwise you would run around or crawl all over the floor of the kitchen, catching and picking up dried out cutouts and yellowed notebook pages covered by different handwriting of women from several generations.

That was precisely the background at the hopeless and obtuse high day of "developed Socialism" (which would later be called "stagnation"),[15] against which the first of W. W. Pokhlebkin's books was perceived. In them he neglected the fetish of "usefulness" and made his credo – tasty cuisine and the return of the happiness of life and the poetry of food. The reader, who had preserved at least a grain of common sense, and who had not been completely fooled by the nonsensical (Soviet-era) "planning" theories, happily responded to his invitation that to "eat" meant to read, to find out, to think, and to cook. Since the time when man invented experimental science, his ability to perceive and understand spreads almost exclusively to his own products, to what he made himself or managed to repeat. Perhaps, that is what Immanuel Kant had in mind when he called everything else the "thing-in-itself."

The second and less significant achievement of Pokhlebkin is an intelligible exposition of the general principles of the kitchen and the meaning of cooking operations, to which the products are subjected in the course of culinary processes. What happens under the lid? Oh, this is an enormous knowledge that frees you, imparts a cook with the power over the still uncooked ingredients of the upcoming dinner, and gives him the necessary freedom for maneuvering and improvising, develops in the kitchen master an intuition similar to that of a composer. It's not in vain that Pokhlebkin compares *"bridost'"* (the term defining the lack of culinary taste which, according to the author, happened because

---

15 A reference to the last decade of Leonid Brezhnev's rule – the 1970s to the early 1980s – known as the period of stagnation.

it was suppressed by the abuse of tobacco and alcohol[16]) to the absence of a musical ear. In his other book, readers were stunned by the description of the cook's tours through famous restaurants, especially because these tours were organized not less pompously than an invitation of famous conductors.

However, any knowledge is a condition that is necessary but not entirely sufficient for cooking success. For example, according to Pokhlebkin, there are 150 types of soups or a thousand variations, including 28 versions of cabbage soup, 22 of borsht, 18 of fish soup, etc., but these are just a classification of groups of food and dishes, similar to that of Linnaeus.[17] There are barely more pure taste sensations, such as "saltiness," "bitterness," "sourness," etc. than the pure colors of the spectrum, but similarly to an artist, who creates his or her own unique color range out of the seven colors of the spectrum (plus black and white), observing and at the same time violating the rules of color interaction (which the almost false science of "color studies" teaches us), the cook, through his or her talent, overarches and remakes our knowledge of taste in his or her own way. And this is Pokhlebkin's third lesson: you need the knowledge in order to neglect it, when necessary; because even the greatest and foundational kitchen principles, without small tricks, or to say it more precisely – intricacies, are nothing but a coarse replica, a dummy of the Soviet Public Food Service homogenization, a universal McDonald's, and, to expand on the point, in the future – chow for astronauts in sealed tubes.

Pokhlebkin's books are well known and constantly reprinted: *Tea, Everything about Spices, The History of Vodka, Mysteries of a Good Kitchen, The Amazing Culinary Art,* or *National Kitchens of Our Peoples* (in which, by the way, perhaps for the first time in our culinary writings he undertook a timid attempt to address some of the

---

16 W. Pokhlebkin *The Secret of a Good Kitchen*.

17 Carl Linnaeus was an 18th-century biologist, the founder of the classification system of species.

mental foundations of the national kitchens, an attempt to describe them as an organic, complex whole, which is inextricably connected with a way for a given people to survive in the concrete historical geographic realia and not always clearly defined predilections. The description of the three waves of influence of the French kitchen on the Russian is simply unforgettable – the influence finally was clarified toward that time as described by Gilyarovsky[18] (however, not for very long as it turned out). The beginning was laid down by the cunning fox Talleyrand,[19] who loaned the best French chef who at his order served the European monarchs, to Alexander I, when the latter came to the Vienna Congress to decide the fate of France after the battle at Waterloo. The art of the great culinary artist Marie-Antoine Careme[20] greatly influenced the mildness of the decision that was accepted by the victors with regard to France. A few years later the first French restaurants opened in St Petersburg and Moscow, and Pushkin belonged to the first generation of Russian gourmets, not just the gastronomes, of the connoisseurs and not simply aficionados. The trophies that the Russian army brought from captured Paris included not only tricks of *amour*, but also new gastronomic notions. But Gogol (perhaps because he was Ukrainian) preferred not the French but the Italian kitchen with its macaroni with marinara sauce and cheese, ravioli, fruit, vegetables, and, possibly, pig lard.

---

18 Vladimir Gilyarovsky was a late nineteenth-century writer and journalist famous for his widely popular description on everyday life in Moscow (street life, trade, restaurants, etc.) in a series of newspaper sketches, published as a book *Moscow and Muscovites* in 1929.

19 Charles Maurice de Talleyrand-Périgord (1754–1838) was a French diplomat in service of Napoleon. However, he betrayed him and dealt with the Russian Tsar Alexander I. After Napoleon's defeat, at the Congress of Vienna in 1814-1815, he negotiated a favorable settlement for France while undoing Napoleon's conquests. He supposedly gave his chef, Marie-Antoine Careme to Tsar Alexander, which resulted not only in the changes in the Russian kitchen but also in favorable outcomes for France at the Congress of Vienna.

20 Marie-Antoine Carême (1784 –1833) was an early practitioner and exponent of the "high art" of French cooking. Carême is often considered one of the first internationally renowned celebrity chefs.

Pokhlebkin's books are "literature" also because they provoke the reader's thought and imagination. His story of how the salt-water frozen fish "gobbled up" the great culinary tradition of cooking fresh-water fish in Russia during the Soviet period, is capable of stirring up emotions to no less of a degree than the drama from the life of Turgenev's dying out nests of gentry.[21] The pictures of the epidemic Russian drunkenness on the eve of the invention of vodka make unexpected corrections to our understanding of Russian history. Pokhlebkin's style, when he goes off the scale, is capable of achieving rare energy. His definition of the porridge cook as a culinary "paramedic" and other similar linguistic gems will be remembered forever.

Nevertheless, they are nothing but linguistic gems because Pokhlebkin has an onerous double. He is also called William Vasilevich Pokhlebkin and he is a professor of history, who wrote a book about vodka at the order of the Kosygin government,[22] a book that is highly interesting but equally biased, and if we argue about superiority in terms of vodka with the Poles about their *gozhalka* (in Ukrainian *horilka*), then you at least have to read it correctly – not like he does it repeatedly – *gorzalka*. He also wrote a lot of works on the history of diplomacy, and the language of the department where he served took vengeance against him, wriggling its way into his books written "for the soul" like the phylloxera, the sap-sucking insect that feeds on leaves and roots of grapevines, and having afflicted his "verbal garden," did not allow him to become a truly great writer.

One of his books simple-heartedly and touchingly reveals before us the drama of a wrong choice: how since his boyhood, enchanted by what was happening in the kitchen, was chased out of there with shouts: "Well you, kitchen commissar, march out of here!" and being called a "girl" even when he just quietly sat in a corner and

---

21 A reference to Ivan Turgenev's novel *A Nest of Gentry* (1859).

22 Aleksei Kosygin was the Chairman of the Council of Ministers, effectively the Prime Minster, of the Soviet Union from 1964 to 1980.

watched. They banished him. There also was the wartime meeting with an amazing army cook, and after the war – university studies and government service. Those whose "spark" was deliberately and for a long time attempted to be extinguished, who studied in Soviet History Departments, who managed to harmonize with the majority of the Party demands in the publishing business – such people often became conscientious government workers.

Pokhlebkin clenched his teeth and quite well managed to do what people wanted and expected from him. But the "spark" eventually caught fire, late, but it caught fire, and "now let everything burn" – the hell with it. As wicked tongues say, it is a gas stove with a torn door that burns with a clear flame at his small, badly equipped kitchen in Podolsk when at the slightest attempt to fire up a burner, a stream of burning gas, like a stream of flame from a flame-thrower, shoots out from the twisted-off handle — how is that not pure literature! Pokhlebkin himself began to resemble a dervish and started to communicate with the world strictly through a post office box.

How Russian all of this is! Even his name – William.

Postscript. In spring 2000 William Pokhlebkin was murdered in his apartment. The killer has not been found to this day. Pokhlebkin's culinary works continue to be reprinted. His seminal work *The Kitchen of the Century*, unprecedented by its historical erudition and the range of his culinary knowledge, came out posthumously. Nowadays Pokhlebkin's works can be found in every big bookstore in Russia. Although the life of the country has drastically changed, the books are still eagerly read. And this is the main sign of classic literature.

In Defense of Sumptuous Eating

Why does the amount of tasteless food constantly increase in the world? You would think that when the iron curtain fell, a gigantic gastronomic world would have opened before us. In comparison with relatively empty store shelves and shameful product "orders" for Soviet holidays (which is sickening to remember, but remember we must), it is true. But the illusion has quickly dissipated. It turned out that the consequence of the lack and over-abundance of provisions results in the development of omnivorousness (not without reason the SU [Soviet Union] and the US [United States] look like an inversion of each other, as one of my American friends has pointed out). Somewhere, as it was in the time of Gilyarovsky, entire fortunes are eaten away through gourmet dinners, but people must have a tightly packed purse, persistency, and know places to do it. Nowadays gourmets have become conspirators and misfits. Some underlying processes force more and more people to eat tasteless and unhealthy food and pay quite a lot for it (which is especially cynical). Nowhere in the world have I met such a great number of unbelievably obese people as in American provincial cities, and I looked at them with a mixture of horror, rapture, curiosity, and repulsion. It would be fine if they ate with delight for the sake of pleasure, but they swallow everything in quick succession in their fast food restaurants with pseudo Chinese and Mexican buffets as well as cheap pizza, chasing everything down with iced drinks at any time of year, turning any food into alimentary garbage with their gluttony.

You can argue about tastes, but fresh oysters "American-style" with ketchup and horseradish (where a humble slice of lemon on ice looks like a relic) is something more than an aberration, it is act of sabotage, an attack on taste receptors and a purposeful obliteration of the very notion of taste. If you look hard, you can find freshly baked bread and soft-boiled potatoes from Idaho, and a suburban store with three thousand sorts of cheese (the French have less than five hundred!), and even a grenade with carcinogens – smoked "kielbasa" (they gave up and introduced the Slavic word into the American dictionary, but nevertheless recommend that it be kept in the freezer), but it doesn't change the fact of the matter. Sooner or later you will give in and start to eat like everyone around you, having completely forgotten about the taste of food: in public fast food places or the ready-made dishes warmed up in the microwave, scrutinizing the labels for the presence of chemicals among the ingredients. It is a universal phenomenon, but particularly in the US, it would seem, that's where the trouble lies. The reason for it is the refusal of much-vaunted individualism and the degradation of home kitchens. If you do not cook (or at least rarely) and only warm up ready-made dishes, atrophy of one of the senses is inevitable. Calorie counts, diets, the tantalizing symbols of exotic kitchens and culinary adventures, and other secondary things will take the place of taste.

Food pluralism is a circular paved road to the wide gates of the universal McDonalds or in Soviet times the *obshchepit* cafeterias. Fortunately, the New Russia is a backward country, where many still believe that food first of all must be tasty, everything else is details.

The Sons of Ursa Major

As I recall, it was the name of a series of children's adventure movies that were shot in East Germany, in which Yugoslav actors[23] played Native Americans. There have been many tribes, dynasties, and cities in the world that have considered bears as their ancestors or patrons. But there has remained one nation that even today is still compared to a bear. Such things, by the way, are not accidental. The dictionary of fauna and flora resembles a code pad on the entrance door: the oak tree is Germany, the rooster is France, the bulldog is England, and the fox is definitely not Russia.

The bear is the most unpredictable animal on account of its thick fir, small ears and short tail (they say that the stubborn bugger is pulled toward honey by the ears and dragged away from it by the tail). For what purpose do they trim the ears and tails of artificial breeds of dogs? So that they obey their master and do not understand each other, like the mute and deaf Gerasim from

---

23 The film was made in 1966 and started an entire series of films about American Indians. Some films were based on the works of James Fenimore Cooper and they starred a Yugoslavian (Serbian) actor Gojko Mitic.

Turgenev's story "Mumu"?[24] After all, it is impossible for them to determine by the wagging of the cut off tail whether it is spit or a kiss, whether you are under attack or your opponent will run away. The Russians don't even argue about the kind of characterization they receive from their neighbors and evil-wishers. There is some truth in it: the largest of the hibernating mammals is moderately lazy, threatening, omnivorous, and human-like. Only the tail-less monkey is more "human-like" than the bear. So, let's bear in mind that in the world of totems, the zodiac, and eastern calendars, all animal symbols are equal and possess equal power. They are distinguished from one another only by their habits, and the result of their competition for a place under the sun more often than not depends on place, time, and luck.

Why do we need all this zoo-philosophy? I answer: it has culinary consequences. I have been wondering for a long time – why the taste receptors of Russian people have not atrophied over the course of several Soviet generations? Why are our people always haunted by a desire to eat something "tasty" or "sweet," and they see food as a holiday and the holiday as an opportunity to eat something otherworldly? Can we forget Ivan Shishkin's painting "Morning in the Pine Forest," the reproduction of which hangs in every other house or the candies called "Misha the Bear in the North?"[25]

Russian hunters divide brown bears into three types: the first includes the largest, carnivorous bovine oppressors (that adore slightly rotten meat) and the Kamchatka lovers of fresh elk meat; the second – lovers of berries and plant roots, hiding in oat fields and raspberry patches; and the third – the smallest, black and malicious

---

24 In Soviet times Ivan Turgenev's short story "Mumu" was widely read in literature courses starting from the middle school to the 10th grade as an example of "critical realism" of the classics of Russian literature. In the story the deaf and mute peasant Gerasim has to drown his beloved dog at the order of a cruel landowner.

25 Ivan Shishkin was a Russian realist painter of the second half of the 19th century. His painting "Morning in the Pine Forest" was indeed one of the three most popular paintings of Russian life. It depicted a family of bears and was used on the wrapper of chocolate candies called "Mishka" (the Bear). The wrapper of "Bear in the North" candy showed a polar bear.

ones with white "bibs" on black fur (until they become mature), the honey lovers and ant-eaters, gourmets *par excellence*.

It would be a sin not to indulge the reader with a recipe of a dish that a hibernating bear may only dream about during long winter months: **ripened raspberry with chilled milk for desert**. *You need to combine raspberries with sugar in a bowl, pour bluish milk over the mixture, and press it down. You can eat it like soup, one that is outrageously tasty, beautiful (the purple in the white), and you will immediately feel sleepy. While bears hibernate and the summer is far away, all that remains for us it is to support ourselves with honey. Bear in mind, honey cannot be kept in the refrigerator or diluted in a cup of hot tea – from the fluctuations in temperature it loses its curative power and turns into just a sweetener. Honey cannot also remain liquid for more than a few months (if it does not thicken, it means that bees were fed sugar) and you can (if not cut it with a knife) spread it over a sweet bun with higher than normal 82.5% sweet cream butter, and wash it down with strong black tea. Do you feel the hot sunny range of different hues, thickness, and temperature?*

Those who doubt it may treat what has been said above as a hypothesis. As for me, I always raise my head at night and first look for the cosmic ladle of Ursula Major, and only after I find it – the axis of the Polar Star.

Tell Me What You Eat…

Somehow we do not exactly realize how much everything is interconnected in the life of individual people and nations. Roughly speaking, if grapes grow well in a particular area, you will drink wine (as done by the French, Italians, Spanish, and others); if the grapes do not grow well or at all, but you do not have problems with grain cultures, it means that you will drink beer (as Germans and the Czechs do) or vodka (as is the case with the Eastern Slavs, who live in a harsher climate). And this is a question of not only the climate and territory, but also culture as a whole where everything is interconnected: the type of housing, the type of behavior, the ways of communication, music, singing, and philosophy. Grossly simplifying, we can say that sausages with beer allow for the appearance of symphonic music, coffee with whipped cream – for the Viennese waltz, while a cup of cooked rice is pregnant with meditation on the sitar. Or it can be the opposite: the symphonic music requires a full dinner, etc. It sounds strange, but try to change anything in these pairs! More so, the neighboring nations living in similar natural climatic conditions in every possible way try to divide into "us" and "not us," and they do this largely through the help of the kitchen.

For example, the three Slavic kitchens – Russian, Ukrainian, and Polish, because of a variety of reasons, are dominated by the inclination towards "sour" cuisine: yeast bread and sour cabbage soups, pickled goods, the role of sour cream (which in Germany, for example, you can find only in Bavaria in the form of their *Schmand*, the rest use *saure Sahne*, that is "sour cream," in reality skimmed off milk that does not have a drop of sourness). But the #1 Russian dish is stewed cabbage soup (it is better if it is made with a beef stock base and half fresh and half sour cabbage, and preferably with a handful of pickled mushrooms). For the Ukrainians it is the scorching hot red borsht with beet tops and slightly undercooked vegetables (the opposite of the Russian kitchen), with grilled root herbs and fixings made out of garlic and grilled lard, rubbed with coarse salt and pepper. The Poles have their stewed *bigos* with the inclusion of all kinds of smoked goods (a German influence) and all kinds of meat, always with prunes. The Russians and Poles also cook and love their red borsht, and Ukrainians and Poles – their own equivalent of cabbage soup, but this fact does not deny the above-mentioned preferences.

The culinary polemics – the extreme dissociation with neighbors and enemies with the help of products and dishes that are unacceptable for them – is even more amusing. Such is historically the case of Ukrainian *salo* (pig lard), which is forbidden for Jews, offensive for the Turks and Tatars (in addition to that, it takes a hell of an effort to rustle the short-legged pig, unlike horses, cattle, or captured people), and for the Russians *salo* is the sign of a settled lifestyle long before the Ukrainians were turned into serfs.[26] But this is a matter of principles; in reality we can see an intense process of borrowing on the edges. The Galicians (the Right-Bank of the Dnipro River Western Ukrainians) successfully mastered shortbreads and hot-cured ring sausages; the Left-Bank Ukrainians – Russian pies; the Southerners adopted the culture of fried food from the Turks, Tatars and Circassians[27] and stopped shunning eggplant; Ukrainian peasants learned from the Jews how to plump up chickens and geese, and Ukrainian city dwellers – how to prepare stuffed and baked fish; Jews, in their turn, learned from the Ukrainians to drink a lot of vodka, chasing it with tender *salo*; and now chefs invited from everywhere to Moscow restaurants prepare Ukrainian borsht with garlic fritters better than ever. That's how it is.

We Do Not Eat It!

I was prompted to think about taste and culinary preferences as one of the most important cultural factors by a conversation I had with my Hutsul[28] friend in the Carpathian Mountains. For the Hutsuls, mushrooms are only the *Boletus* (White Mushroom), the rest are "mushroom relatives": *kozari* (birch boletus and red-cap boletus), *yashnitsi* (variegated boletus), *lisitsi* (literally: foxes; chanterelle), *pidpenki* (string mushrooms), and *golubinki* (Russula mushrooms) – here the edible mushrooms end, which, by the way, shows that the Hutsuls are an ecdemic people who are not forest natives, even if they have been living there for more than a thousand years. I was

---

26 Ukrainian peasants were made serfs (that is, "attached" to the land owned by landowner and thus the latter's property) by Catherine II's decree of 1773.

27 Circassians are an ethnic group in the North Caucasus Mountains region.

28 Hutsuls are colorful inhabitants of the Carpathian Mountains in Western Ukraine.

charmed by the simplicity of this formula: "We know that there are other edible mushrooms, but we, the Hutsuls, do not eat them." Another thought: the Hutsuls, with their sheep flocks and subalpine meadows, and Bukovynian Moldovans[29] could produce not only wonderful sheep milk feta cheese but also the hard cheeses that wouldn't be any worse than those of the Swiss. It, of course, would require enormous efforts, but the question here is, wouldn't they then cease to be Hutsuls and Moldovans in the process?

Let's then consider more closely the difference between Russians and Ukrainians. It would seem that you cannot find peoples closer than these two.

The Ukrainians did not consider beef as meat because oxen were used for plowing and pulling of carts, and cows – for producing milk, while for the Russians it has been a primary meat dish. The Russians are not against pork, but it must be lean and without lard, without which the Ukrainians cannot even imagine their life. If you remove *salo* from their diet, a huge number of Ukrainian dishes, including deserts, simply could not be prepared, and the Ukrainians might be easily confused with Turks or Crimean Tatars.

At the same time both the Russian and Ukrainian kitchens grew out of the same root. This is the common source of the lively sourness of rye bread, yeast dough, and not the Asian flatbread; bread or beet *kvas*, pickled and not marinated vegetables, and the preferential place of soups in the menu, which the Russian appropriately call the "first course." The Russians and Ukrainians equally value the sweet-and-sour taste, but the Russian also succeeded in making so-called sweet-and-sour "take-the-hair-off-the dog" soups: *solyanka* (spicy vegetable and meat soup), *rassolnik* (pickled cucumber soup), *kalya* (cucumber brine soup), and others. Despite the fact that the Russians mastered and included red borsht in their menu, and the Ukrainians borrowed meat pies from the

---

[29] Bukovyna (Bucovina in Romanian) is a historical region divided nowadays between Ukraine and Romania. It is located on the northern slopes of the Carpathian Mountains.

Russians, serious differences in cooking principles have remained. The Russians stew their soups and prefer simmering and baking as dictated by the Russian stove. The Ukrainians, on the contrary, value undercooked vegetables in their soups and necessarily add sautéed vegetable roots to them. The Turks turned out to be better teachers of frying food than the Tatars for the Russians. The Ukrainians also borrowed the idea of their *varenyky* (dumplings; especially with cottage cheese and cherries) from the same Turks, as the Russians – their idea of Siberian *pelmeni* (meat dumplings) from the Komi people living around today's city of Perm. The Ukrainians contrived to add cottage cheese to the dough to make it more tender, the Russians – sour cream. The Ukrainians more often than the Russians use unleavened dough (from the *halushki* [unstuffed dumplings] to sweet pastries). Both peoples like kashas (porridges), but for the Russian the first place among them is occupied by buckwheat groats (even Russian *bliny* require buckwheat flour), while for the Ukrainians, first place belongs to millet (to prepare the famous Cossack *kulesh* (thin gruel), millet was fried with pig lard before a campaign, and the only thing required to eat it was to add water and boil it. (The original way, by the way, which used to stun foreigners but is now forgotten by many other peoples, was – to throw scorching hot stones into a pot).

By way of illustration, let me provide a table of priorities in the respective Russian and Ukrainian kitchens:

Russian Kitchen	Ukrainian Kitchen
cabbage soup	borsht
beef	pork
jellied or aspic meat	jellied pigs feet
pelmeni (meat dumplings)	varenyky (potato, cottage cheese or cherry dumplings)
buckwheat	millet
baked meat or fish pies	small fried pies
bliny (crepe-like thin pancakes)	olad'i (thick, medium size pancakes)
prostokvasha (curdled milk)	ryazhenka (fermented baked milk)

eggs sunny-side-up	scrambled eggs or omelet
white cabbage	beets with tops
potatoes	legumes and beans
cucumber	tomato
dill weed	lovage (parsley)
apples	prunes
raspberries	cherries (that is why Anton Chekhov's play Cherry Orchard that is set in the south of Russia was perceived as "non-Russian" and outraged the Northerner Ivan Bunin)
jam	marmalade

Many names of Ukrainian dishes, thanks to Nikolai Gogol's good graces, sound so appetizing to the Russian ear that it seems you can eat them: *pechenya, vereshchaka, shpundra, zavyvanets, verguny, or pukhkenyky.*

It goes without saying that the Russian kitchen is richer and more diverse, and the Ukrainian more monolithic. If we look for an analogy, the Russian kitchen differs from the Ukrainian approximately in the same way as the French (and the French worked quite a bit on improving the Russian table in the 19th century) from the Italian (with its less refined but more compelling peasant southern taste). It is not an accident that Pushkin adored French restaurants that opened in the capitals, and Gogol ran away from Petersburg to Rome where he went crazy over macaroni and cheese, which upon his return to Russia he himself used to cook and treat his Moscow friends.

PART II
Cultural Dictionary of Eastern Slavic Food

Salo (Pig Lard)

To M. Epshtein[30]:
Ukrainianness, Russianness, Sovietness

1. Does a cuisine have anything to do with a certain nation's fate, with a mindset, a philosophy?

Only a hopelessly narrow mind would answer this question in the negative. Nevertheless, we usually imply that there is such a connection, but do not comprehend it. Why is that so? Is it the result of the nearsightedness of our sense of touch, of smell, and of taste overcome by longer-range sight and hearing? There is no doubt about it either. The human larva drags everything into its mouth, and this stage settles deep down somewhere at the foundation of an adult whose senses are determined by the primacy of sight and hearing and by the suppression of cannibalism.

How many words do we have in our culture to designate taste? Sour, sweet, salty, bitter, tart, "tasty" – that's about it. It is truly the vocabulary of a primate. However, one of the wildest mysteries of a refined intuitive culture is called transubstantiation and communion. There is apparently something fundamental in the sensation of taste repressed by a rationalistic culture, something that pierces through all levels of humanity in a human being and protrudes somewhere… into nowhere. One can eat one's fill and belch, one can "*napertysia horniatkom kashi*" (eat till you burst), one can feast or indulge in the culinary art of food and drink, but – eliminating avarice – we will be interested only in satisfying hunger, in fortifying one's strength. Why does the presently anecdotal (and deserving of special interest), mythic *SALO* (incredibly edible PIG LARD) appear as so much the quintessence

---

30 Mikhail Epstein is a Russian thinker and literary-philosophy scholar. He is founder and director of the Centre for Humanities Innovation at Durham University and the author of *The Transformative Humanities: A Manifesto* (New York–London, 2012). He and Klekh are close friends.

of Ukrainian ethnic culture? What kind of product is it and what does it contain?

2. Pig lard for Ukrainians is the same as Manna for the Jews (and the apples of Hesperides[31] for the Greeks), that is, a transcendental and earth-shattering dish, and for differentiation (as they say "out of spite" or to have them in "spades") from the neighbors to the South, the Judeo-Muslims, it is undoubtedly prohibited for *them*.[32] It is a dish that is both public and sacred, polemically sharpened. Consuming it resembles gliding on skis.

In the world of perishable products in the South, it is non-perishable and in some way the equivalent of gold. It comprises the cult of abundance that originates in the fat pagan gods of happiness, Biblical pomace, and also the dry Cossack ration, emergency stores of the poor, sprinkled with the thick salt of the Chumak road.[33] In its taste you can distinctly feel echoes of that Chumak road – whether it is because people take it with them for a trip, or because *salo* calls for a long journey along beaten down, opened up Ukrainian "*shlyakhy*" (dirt roads), drowning in soft white road dust like the Milky Way.

From those carts, the axles, the leather boxes filled with lard to grease the axles, the far-reaching wisdom of the first social mechanisms is drawn – "if you don't grease up, you won't go." And from the same source comes the specifically Ukrainian word "sum" [pronounced "soom"], the sadness of a traveler sitting by the side of the road (because "*sadlo*," the original form of the word "*salo*," is something that has settled down, packed down on meat, and from the same root come the words "session" [*sessiia*] and "conference"

---

31 In Greek mythology, the Hesperides are nymphs who tend a magical apple orchard in the far west corner of the world.

32 Klekh is playing with words here: "to spite" in the Russian original is "v piku," which literally means "to play a spade." The original for "prohibitive" is an adjective "trefnoe," which refers to food proscribed in the Jewish faith, but it also is associated with the playing card suit of clubs.

33 The *chumak* was a Ukrainian oxcart driver, who transported grain to Crimea and brought back salt, fish, and other goods. Klekh is also playing here on the Ukrainian phrase for the Milky Way "Chumatskyi shliakh."

[*zasedanie*]...), yes, of the traveler who has lost his way and is sitting now under the boundless sky, under the clouds, that lard of the heavens. To accompany it, a *tsybulyna* (an onion) is procured and cut into four parts, which eases the welling of tears of the sad high *priest* who has found himself far from home.

It is a universal product that gives light, when it is melted down for an oil lamp or in the shape of a tallow candle. It is dreadfully rich in calories, when it is cut off with a knife in a thin "*skibochka*" (sliver). Its assimilability is traced even in the phonetic form of its name – the gliding "S" and the moist, deglutitive "L" – and the vowels AO. The salted lard, bittersweet onion, "*horilka*" (home-brewed Ukrainian vodka), unleavened bread slightly oxidized with saliva – in a wide-open field – that is, the fundamental meal of the steppe-living Slav. At the sight of such a scene, pride grows in the heart, the way lard grows on a pig.

3. (In sum) *Vazhko vtrymatys', aby ne skazaty: "salo – nashe use"* (If we think about it, how can we not say that "for us *salo* is everything"?)

The *Blin*

A blin *won't harm your stomach.*
V. Dal'[34]

If you project the cross section of the world tree onto Russian cuisine, you will get a *blin* (a pan-fried flat cake something like a crepe).

You can find one of the most unique cosmogonic myths in a Russian fairytale about an old woman who was cooking *bliny* on the baldpate of her not-getting-any-younger husband. With the use of solar energy, of course.[35] Generally speaking, the echoes of the solar

---

34 V. Dal', *Poslovitsy i pogovorki russkogo naroda* (Proverbs and Sayings of the Russian People).

35 A reference to a Russian folktale about a woman married to the sun, which cooked *bliny* on his head.

origin of *bliny* are clear even for us who do not believe in anything. After all, the shape of a circle is not at all simpler than, let's say, that of a triangle, and the matter here is not limited by economy alone.

Cooking is one of the most ancient of theatrical performances, especially in the case of basic dishes prepared with a minimum of means: flour, water, and fire. And a little bit of oil, of course.

The most Russian aspect of making *bliny* is that it comprises an exciting activity when it is going well and one can ignore the law of "the first blin."[36] This way there appear constellations of pancakes; the chthonic *deruny* (potato pancakes); barley, wheat, oat, and buckwheat *bliny*; *bliny* from leavened and yeast dough, with all kinds of stuffing and without; tiny oily pancakes, hotcakes, and flapjacks. Generally speaking, tea drinking with *bliny* from a samovar is nothing else but a model of the universe, a national Russian planetarium where the cups and saucers are Saturns and Plutos following their orbits, and the scalding hot tea is analogous to life-giving sunlight, which, by the way, the resourceful Russians learned to catch and deposit in the yellow of butter and honey.

But the *bliny* take their most intense form at wakes where *bliny* with caviar are served first. Hot *bliny* with chilled caviar are both an inversion and a shroud that conceal the hyperbole of cornucopia. Death pregnant with life. In light of what has been said above, the monopoly of the privileged classes and the state trade on the sale of caviar appears as nothing else but a symbolic usurpation of the right of the powerful, one for the continuation of the species.

Without penetrating the consciousness and self-realization of the people, in the waning days of the *stagnation* during the Brezhnev era this thought spilled into a collective madness over UFOs – when the tired, hungry, and ill-fed raised their heads and suddenly saw still hot *bliny* flying over them. The outrageous thing about them was that it was very difficult to establish contact with

---

36 A reference to a Russian saying "The first *blin* always comes out crooked," meaning "better luck next time" or "you must spoil before you spin."

them. But this also inspired a belief that sooner or later the people will get to them.

That was how the preconditions of [Mikhail Gorbachev's liberalization policy of] *perestroika* came about. Interestingly enough almost simultaneous to the information about the UFOs, a new Russian swearword appeared – "Bli-n-n-n!"[37] – like a resounding slap on the face, like an American pie in the face.

It was then that the Party understood that *perestroika* could no longer be postponed.

Kielbasa as a Political Measure

As it was discovered, negative and even imaginary measures exist in the material world, too. One such measure is kielbasa.

Mistaken are those who think that this measure is dominant and serves digestion—not at all. It is called upon to satisfy not hunger (because there has been no hunger in the USSR for a long time), but the libido. The proof of this is the fact – and it is its main characteristic – that there is always either no kielbasa or not enough of it in the stores. Metaphysics shines and sparkles through its physical nature and the psychic mist that envelops it. Most likely, kielbasa indeed represents that phosphorescent, substantially deceptive phallus by means of which the Party accomplishes its proclaimed unity with the people.

Perestroika revealed this hidden nature of kielbasa particularly clearly. When several prominent [in the dual sense] *members* (*chleny*) of the [feminine in gender] Party (*Partiya*) died and she stopped screwing the populace (*narod*) [masculine in gender] through all nine of his orifices, and having begun to intensely titillate the head of her own clitoris, with only five of the orifices remaining, the populace all of a sudden rose up and, upon seeing that the Party did not love it as much as she-it once did, suddenly

---

37 A reference to the Russian swear word "blin," which is a euphemism for "blyad'" (which literally means "slut," but whose closest English equivalent is "crap.")

came to their senses and angrily demanded kielbasa, threatening a divorce otherwise. No matter how much the Party strained all its Fallopian tubes for the next five years, nothing came out of them except for *glasnost*.[38]

We just point out to skeptics that the people demand kielbasa – not meat, not content! – but form. The evidence of this consists of successful experiments with the substitution of meat in kielbasa stuffing with wood pulp, as a result of which the lines for kielbasa – this political guarantee of love – only grew longer. A love-deprived people behave like a child looking for punishment – going to the extreme of permissiveness in search of punishment – and despite all his tears, feeling relief from a symbolic spanking at their mother's hand or from the belt in their father's hand, which, in the end, saves him from himself. The ontological roots of kielbasa go deep into the human makeup, into both of man's intestinal tracts: the one in the brain and the other in the stomach, which are ideally accommodated: the first – for the cognition of the idea of kielbasa, the second – for the consumption of its body. Is it worthwhile to elaborate that such consumption represents an act of sexual-political cannibalism?

Generally speaking it must be pointed out that the erotic nature of kielbasa is of a universal and complex character. We can single out some of its aspects as voyeuristic, others as oral, and all the way to the fecal – the eating of the contents of the intestines (which, by the way, has been understood by the people by bringing together the sound of the word "*kal*" (feces) with the word "*kolbasá*" [pronounced *kalbasá*]. It is obvious that the richness and diversity of experiences infinitely deepen and broaden the mindset of any people, which periodically has to deal with the issue of kielbasa, it

---

38   Klekh is playing with the gender of these various word forms in Russian, seeing the Communist Party (*partiia*), as feminine in gender, but with *chleny* (members; i.e., having members/penises). In Klekh's verbal mythology, the *narod*, the populace, which is masculine in gender, was constantly being screwed by the feminine in gender party. He also astutely observes that the Politburo consisted of nine members (pun intended), the same as the number of orifices in the human body.

places such a people on the threshold of a sixth sense discovered by Socialism, a sense of deep satisfaction, where the people and Socialism, once having met, never part from each other. It also seems to be significant that yet at the dawn of our century, the century of the victorious march of the ideas of the Great October Socialist Revolution, kielbasa, particularly in its Russian pronunciation "*kal-ba-sá*," became a part of international Esperanto.

And that future is not far off, that hour, that realization of the bright hallucinations of mankind, when well-ordered KIELBASA as such, liberated from individual names and misdescription, will be coiled onto spools for telephone cables and delivered to grocery stores by trucks similar to fire engines in order to be fed like a hose, like a beating and pulsating fire truck intestine, to an entire line of people, to complete and final satiety.

Vodka as Pure Alcohol

There are people who say you shouldn't drink. They are under the influence for their entire life from birth. You can always strain off a glass of dry wine from the blood of any abstinent. The discoverer of the caves with Ideas[39] used to say that till a certain age you shouldn't drink at all, then – moderately, after 40 – definitely. And go dancing. That's how it was supposed to be in his Ideal State.

Many people have written about drinking. Intoxication is glorified. But even our cookbooks remain silent about vodka as an ingredient. Its consequences are always present and obvious, its essence, however, is as elusive as… I don't remember what it's called. There are other drinks that exist for your pleasure. Wine has flavor that can be better or worse. Vodka doesn't have any flavor: it only has potency. In Russian vodka this potency is established at an optimal point – at an abyss, at the fortieth degree longitude lies the capital of a state called Alcohol. Mendeleev's undergraduate work on water-soluble spirits did nothing else but confirm the correctness

---

39 A reference to Plato's *Republic*.

of the intuition of the people who forever linked their fate to… fire, water, and copper tubing.[40]

The apparatus for distilling spirits was invented a thousand years ago by Arab alchemists; in order to bypass the religious prohibition, they created something that didn't exist, but who remembers that now?

In Russia to drink is a matter of honor, conscience, and reason.

Vodka represents man's true and sole drinking companion. Through vodka he realizes his union with the elements: water, fire, grain that comes from the earth, and… *spirit* extracted from the pores of this world. Vodka – also called *gorelka* (burner), *gor'kaia* (bitter), *palenka* (fire-water), by its appearance is indistinguishable from water (and, after all, you must drink water, pure as a tear, but 40° proof!). But in the world of drinks, vodka – just as at a feast of cold steel arms – is a double-edged sword that has no name. Nourishing, it sets one's blood on fire and rises in a person as a categorical imperative, and very few mortals can meet the burden of the demands it makes. Roughly speaking, a few know how to drink. Vodka turns a person's insides out, making the hidden manifest for a single evening. That's why hypocrites don't like it so much, as well as some other people who resemble, say, flat-bottomed boats.

The sister of a philosopher – more than two thousand years ago Greeks would allow themselves to dilute wine with water – has in fact nothing to say to people: it is empty like the vacuum of space, it is only a hand-mirror placed before lips, the horror of a zombie – are you sure that the mirror will be covered with mist this time?

The Metaphysics of a Hangover

The weakening of the force of gravitation during drinking intensifies the force of gravitation during a hangover. The tongues of alcohol that lick your veins turn out to be the cold hellish flame

---

40 A Russian saying "to pass fire, water, and copper tubing" which means "to pass the hardest test" or "to survive the most terrible ordeal."

of a hangover under your skull, when your entire body labors like a smoking stove overstuffed with wet logs, with your abominably healthy heart knocking around in your chest like a traitor.

Drunkenness burned up the oxygen under the suffocating cap of the sky – it is not even enough oxygen for the unsealed letters of Hypnosis – without an address and unstamped – that were placed on your head like compresses since the night, to smolder and shrivel up (if not even burn up completely).

O, canine world made of papier-mâché! – the poverty of self-recognition that long ago deduced the futility of coitus, but nevertheless keeps asking to go out like a child in kindergarten – to go pee-pee. And the stench comes out of your mouth as though you had buried someone inside you.

And this crudeness of earthly alcohol that is *spirit* only in name is just a linguistic mistake!

All things in the world suddenly lose their meaning as if a snapshot had captured them. Which residue that doesn't settle out as any kind of sediment did you look for at the bottom of your imagination? Why and how, having traversed the narrow and tense path of anxiety, having accomplished a successful escape from the world of numbing worries, you suddenly came to your senses all covered with slimy clay, as if in an Asian earthen prison pit?

After all it not always was like that – there were times of blurriness of vision when the next day you drank more than the night before and an ordinary kitchen table set for breakfast suddenly became transformed: steam rose from a coffee cup like dust from suede in a beam of sunlight stretching from the sky; on that table the most common objects were scattered in disarray, but your hands did not wander around, building perpendicular-parallel rows of matches relative to the edge of the table and the pattern on the table-cloth, and placing a fork – relative to the food: and where a finch – perhaps, a distant offspring of the one about which Pushkin spoke in his next to last poem – sang when it wanted to.[41]

---

41 A reference to a pseudo-children's song attributed to Alexander Pushkin "Finch-

And under the window a girl could walk along the vacant lot – she was walking! – do you remember?... crows were not afraid of her though she had a stick in her hand, she broke ice on frozen puddles with it; a little back and to the side of her, an empty plastic bag that looked like a little dog skipped along the hillocks; every minute the girl bent over something, thumped and dug into something with her stick until it broke, and then she ran in the direction of the road where a bus was already turning around, with her backpack and a bag with her school uniform swinging left and right, making her run herky-jerky and off balance....

"Expand on your thought, expand on it!" Your drinking buddies shouted to you the night before. All your life you have waited for signs, winding up time onto yourself with a winch in order to pull up your cage closer to death.

All the tasty things have already been eaten.

Your bread from now on is like dry excrement, and your drink – like sealed bile. The "wheels" are powerless.

There is no path leading out of this feverish Devonian forest, invisible for those who live in ultraviolet light... Who? Silence.

Hell! I am your victory.

But your hour is not yet today. It has not yet chimed.

Once again it rises up, and I don't know what to do with it.

The ambulance of the typewriter carriage rushes in toward the beginning of a new paragraph, saving your life.

Soup Therapy

Strictly speaking, what is the cause of people getting sick and dying? Not because of infections per se, but because they gave in to the infection because their immunity had weakened, their aura had holes in it, their skin had become thinner – you look and see that it

---

Pinch, where've you been?/ – I was drinking vodka on Fontanka Street...," and more precisely to his 1836 poem "Having forgotten the grove and freedom,/ An accidental finch above me/ Pecks at the grain and splashes water,/ And amuses itself with a lively song."

is already not a person lying on a hospital bed – the next thing for him is to kick the bucket. But I am not talking about a bad ending, I am talking about a good start.

I was always struck by the fact that common people and people of the older generation always try to feed a sick person, even against his or her will. Or another example: they get on a train and immediately begin to eat – they take out a whole chicken or homemade cutlets, cut tomatoes in half, etc. Now I understand – how simple it is! Our body is a house, our stomach is a stove; the home has to be warmed up, no one will live in a chilly house. The food is not just calories, but it is also materialized care, the simple-hearted and awkward care of loved-ones when we talk about sick people. By the way, for those who do not know it, our human kiss originates in the symbolic ritual of feeding that people saw in birds (among many other things such as our dances and singing, navigation and aviation), and those who did not see it well, rub their noses against each other, but there are very few of those.

At this point I would like to sing the praises of concentrated chicken bouillon because there is nothing better than it for strengthening someone, who is ill. But…! First of all, there are almost no properly fed chickens left in our urbanized world, and second, we have the bird flu that came to replace mad cow disease, so be sure to look for the right chicken!

I limit myself to giving praise to borsht. When the flu season is just around the corner or you experience the unpleasant sensations of a virus you caught somewhere, put all your errands aside and stand by the stove to cook a big pot of borsht. Color is the principle here – hot, scorching, fiery red, the color of summer. It is worth preparing borsht even during Lent, let those who observe it forgive me. Because, first of all, not everyone observes Lent; secondly, the church gives dispensations to those who take ill; and thirdly, nothing stops you from making borsht out of dry "white" Boletus mushrooms (which undoubtedly represents the Ukrainian contribution in the recipe of borsht), and as for the "non-Lenten color" – you cannot do anything about it, but, honest to God, what

Russian does not like this as one of the most beautiful dishes in the world? I know a lot of people who, as soon as they go to live abroad, begin to cook borsht – the name itself – isn't it something!

If you visit a sick person in a hospital,[42] you should bring just the broth in a thermos, and then add chopped dill to the cup. The rich but not greasy bouillon with a neutral taste and tender aroma is capable of, if not bringing the sick person back from the underworld, then returning to him or her a taste for life in any case.

The Invention of Cheese

In the dictionary of Vladimir Dal,[43] there is a saying, in which a subliminal longing for cheese is placed on record: "I don't eat raw food, I don't want fried, I can't stand boiled." As in the Russian fairytale: "Go there, I don't know where, bring that, I don't know what."[44] Neither raw nor boiled cheese represents this intermediate product, of which it is hard to say where it comes from (though cheese makers prepare it at cheese factories). After all, in the beginning was milk. Turning sour, it became unsuitable for use, worthless – like man after the fall from grace. And suddenly from this essentially spoiled liquid people extracted and built an entire sour-milk world, introducing a delectable chapter to the history of the culinary art. As bad as we might be in many other aspects, with a thought about cheese and several other achievements of civilization, I am personally puffed up with pride and wonder. We can understand how cottage cheese is made out of curdled milk; how the Central Asian *suzma* (the milk product that stands between cottage cheese and sour cream) is made out of *qatiq* (natural yoghurt); or ricotta – from whey; but it is not so easy do with

---

42   In Russia relatives and friends normally bring food to patients since the hospitals in general do not provide cafeteria services.

43   Vladimir Dal was the author of the famous *Explanatory Dictionary of the Living Great Russian Language*, which was published between 1863-1866.

44   A fixed phrase that gives instructions to the hero for his quest.

porous Swiss cheese, that has come about as the result of a calf's gizzard dropped into yeast, or the rotting Roquefort, developing from cheese mold! Those who love just unsavory "Russian" cheese or sweet vanilla-flavored cottage cheese in chocolate would never understand that. I remember with what contempt the Soviet people standing in a customary store queue stared at the capital weirdoes, who preferred rank Roquefort at 2 rubles 50 kopecks to the Russian "Rossiisky cheese" at 2 rubles 70 kopecks per kilogram, which could be so nicely placed on an open-faced sandwich with butter for a spot of tea that came from a box with a little elephant on the label[45] (there were, I remember, also Kostroma, Uglich and Bukovyna cheeses,[46] and when they didn't come out right for the manufacturing technicians, they would become *Poshekhonsky* cheese [a sort of Russian "redneck" cheese]), because they all were sold unripened; keeping them in the refrigerator appreciably made their taste better, which even today, by the way, would not harm many different kinds of cheese). In those store lines I learned the best definitions of socialism – that is the absence of variety: instead of different kinds of food products, we had generic "fish," "meat," "cheese," "macaroni." When we reached the all-encompassing concept of "food" in our generalizations, socialism kicked the bucket before the population did it.

I must admit, I have no particularly deep affection for the French, but I love their cheeses and wines – and de Gaulle, exclaiming in a fit of rage: "How can you govern a people that has 379 different kinds of cheese?!" I don't need that many but if I don't have at least twenty, life would be no joy for me. In my brain there is a small cheese pedestal: the king and champion is Roquefort, the real thing, and not its imitation "Dor Bleu," forgive me Lord; the silver medal goes to a wedge of parmesan (and the older it is, like a callous on

---

45   A reference to so-called "Indian Tea" that was extremely popular in Soviet times.

46   The cities of Kostroma and Uglich were two major cheese-producing centers in the Volga region in Russia. Bukovina is an area in Western Ukraine famous especially for production of feta-type cheeses.

your heel, the harder and yellower it is); the bronze would go to Swiss Gruyere and Emmentaler; fourth place to the fat and crumbly *brynza* (Georgian feta cheese). As in any real competition, at times they change rankings, but they never sink lower than fifth place. It's better to cut up hard cheeses into a thick straw. And brine cheeses, even the royal Bulgarian cow feta is tastiest with hot hard-boiled polenta (Italian grits) and tomatoes without salt (in the winter use only cherry tomatoes). It's too bad to part with you, dear reader, without these simple suggestions.

"Say – Che-e-ese!"

Hangover Cookery

The regrettable condition of a hangover is a weighty argument, but of a lower order to use as a refusal from abusing alcohol. A certain psychiatrist, my childhood friend, advised everyone to reject occasional shameful drunkenness, which leads to pseudo-binge-drinking (when one drinks not from an internal need, but "for company"), but instead of this load up on alcohol twice a month, so that you maintain a healthy psyche. He proscribed his personal abstinence syndrome with followers of his teachings at weekly Saturday soccer matches and the bathhouse with beer after that. A certain part of his advice sank into my soul, as happens in youth, and allowed me over time to accumulate my personal practical experience.

We'll leave the metaphysical, psychological, and social bases for the abuse of alcohol aside (and this, undoubtedly, is an indecisive and semi-conscious form of suicidality), concentrating exclusively on the corporeal aspect and on what one can undertake, in order to emerge from a critical condition that gives you an idea of what it would feel like being in hell (where the church, not without reason, places drunkards).

Of course, "an active life" is always preferable, i.e., soccer (or skiing) and a sauna afterward, but if this for some particular reason is impossible or turns you off too much (resources for self-restraint aren't unlimited), one can try a softer variant and strive to return to normal life activity through the kitchen. Work therapy that does not demand a certain amount of super effort is not only inevitable, but also desired. The fulfillment of compulsory service in the kitchen has as its nearest goal to make up for the organism's deficiency of those nourishing and mineral substances and vitamins that the alcohol burned and washed out. The organism must not *give to drink*, but *to nourish* (therefore the inordinate use of liquid the next day is the most widespread mistake; after all an alcoholic is a person, who has shifted to liquid products for nourishment, calories in pure form, which alcohol supplies; they are more easily digested, and the organism, always inclined to laziness, unnoticeably falls in this way into biochemical dependence).

You can begin by making a non-alcoholic cocktail, from time immemorial called **"The Morning of Our Homeland"**: *into a tart tomato sauce (or tomato paste with ajika[47] or salt and pepper) squeeze a clove of garlic through a garlic press, then add – mandatorily, and this is the main nuance! – minced green dill or several drops of essence of dill, you drop in an entire egg yolk, and this entire mixture is shaken and churned up in a bottle (preferably a glass one) of mineral water. The bursting little bubbles and the yellow luminary floating up over the bloody-red horizon, which you swallow and which slips down your alimentary canal, along with other teasing and refreshing ingredients will be the thing that eventually will bring you to your senses.*

Only just such a cocktail prepared according to the recipe that has been carefully passed down from generation to generation, from hand to hand, has the right to be called "The Morning of Our Homeland," and not the odious inventions of boozers, abstractionists "in life."

Thirst isn't a fancy, and you should remember that no amount of water will quench it. Fermented or sour milk (*katyk*) is better.

---

47 A hot, spicy Georgian sauce.

Of the brines, a cabbage one is considered the best for the simple reason that strictly speaking, it is cabbage juice and not water, like the one added during the pickling process to cucumbers and tomatoes. If you do not have any kind of brine, you shouldn't try to replace it with marinades – this is a perilous path of imitating our "younger brothers in reason," who try without thinking anything that is nearby in the futile hope that it will give them relief. Not too bad in terms of a first step would be about three glasses of a strong freshly brewed piping hot tea with lemon and sugar, which will give a shock-inducing dose of mysterious life-giving vitamin C and tannins to your organism.

In order to dispose your organism toward egress from the hangover (and in any case, not to allow yourself to slip inadvertently back into a drinking binge), it is necessary to firmly and in a variety of ways nourish it. You can step out to the nearest market and buy groceries, catching a breath of fresh air while doing that, and immediately indulge yourself in the preparation of food. Whatever you happen to make, from boiled potatoes to fried eggs with *salo* or bacon, all will be good. A hot soup, that would extract from vegetables, chicken, or anything you want those nourishing substances that are so necessary for your life would be even better. The more concentrated the dish is (not containing more ingridients!), the better. After the first scorching spoonfuls, you'll immediately break into a sweat. Now, accompanied by the hot dish, you can finally drink a glass of vodka (we are talking here about the traditional variety of hangover, specific to our climate; a wine hangover is greatly helped by chilled oysters with champagne, but even to mention similar methods of sobering up in mass-market writing would be simply cynical).

Everything that I mentioned, however, has, strictly speaking, nothing to do with hangover cookery. Hot first courses are distinctly divided into two basic types. The first is the classic line of sour Russian soups: *shchi, rassolniki* and *solyanki* of all different types (their distinguishing characteristic is that you always have them at hand in the refrigerator, you can eat them cold, without putting it off for a long time; and later, after you have gained your strength and put yourself together, you can gobble up a small warmed-up bowl).

The opposite trend consists of thick, colloidal, jelly-like cold soups and dishes of a southern and, partly, Central-European origin (the Caucasian *khash* or *khashi*, the Western Slavic *flyachky*, that is specially prepared tripe. They are eaten only piping hot.

From the first type, so-called rich or full *shchi* are the most preferable and also the fish *solyanka*. The ingredients of full *shchi* include:

>**meat with bone** *(cook no less than two hours at the lowest possible temperature in an uncovered pot with root greens and bay leaf);*
>
>**a mixture of pickled and chopped fresh cabbage**, *which is stewed in a deep covered stewing pot, in a small quantity of water with a tablespoon of butter, and then is added into the prepared strained meat bouillon; in which the diced potatoes had been boiled first (to avoid hardening in the acid environment), and only after that the stewed cabbage is added;*
>
>**green roots** *(which, if you can't tolerate the taste of boiled onions, are better sautéed on a frying pan in vegetable oil);*
>
>**mushrooms** *(you can use dried ones previously soaked in water, but much better marinated, and even better – both, as they say, you won't spoil kasha with butter, even more so because the consistency, taste and aroma of them are different);*
>
>*don't spare* **bay leaves** *(one leaf per plate), pepper (ten or so crushed black peppercorns or a piece of paprika), and at the very end add several cloves of crushed garlic.*
>
>*If you're not lazy, then get the shchi to an unparalleled stewed taste best of all in an oven – in an earthenware pot, a thick-walled pot, or if worse comes to worst, in a metallic pot without plastic handles or even in an enamel roasting pan. Let the combined ingredients stew at least for a half hour to an hour at a moderate temperature (200-300° F). After portioning out the thick shchi into bowls, return the earthenware metallic*

pot with the remaining shchi to the oven to slowly cool in it (in this way the prepared shchi won't lose its taste over the following days). Dissolve a Tbsp of sour cream into the bowls and sprinkle chopped up greens on top, which will soften the taste and will add a whiff of freshness to the dish. This is it concerning shchi.

Solyanka, especially the fish version of it, is associated by most with a restaurant menu, though preparing it is very uncomplicated and for any family supper will add a festive tonality.

Either slightly salted or fresh red fish go into it (from loach (Arctic salmon) and hunchback salmon to Atlantic salmon, sockeye salmon and nova salmon), and even better – two types together. From fresh fish, the ideal is the head of Atlantic salmon, by virtue of the presence of cartilage and gum substances and tender cuts, which, when cooked, resemble a soufflé. For the fish bouillon to turn out concentrated – this is what the taste of the future solyanka depends on – I would recommend taking apart a partially cooked fish on a cutting board, not even very thoroughly, the meatiest parts, after that – the backbone, bones of the head (the gills should be removed even earlier during the cutting!), return the tail and fins to an open pot to boil with roots and spices (celery is much preferred – either the roots or leaves). After an hour the bouillon, cooked on low, and reduced approximately in two, will just need to be strained through a cheesecloth or colander.

In the meantime, in a deep stewing pan or frying pan, sauté pickles, chopped up in small cubes in their own brine, and olives in a ladle of fish bouillon, if they're not sufficiently tender. You can also add skinned tomatoes (to take the skins off easily, drop the tomatoes for several seconds into the nearby boiling fish bouillon). In the absence of tomatoes to give a specific taste to the sour environment, and also for color, you'll also need to add to the solyanka a few Tbsps of tomato paste, otherwise the color of the prepared dish will turn out to be dirty-brown, which will be quite unappetizing to look at, and the taste obviously will *also be lacking something. Separately you should sauté the roots and stalks of greens in vegetable oil.*

After that the strained concentrated bouillon is combined with the stewed salted vegetables, and the sautéed and partly cooked boned fish, chopped up into small pieces. Some love to use pickled cabbage instead of salted pickles, or in addition to them, in their solyanka, but in that case it would be worthwhile to cut the cabbage up with a knife crosswise so it doesn't hang over from the spoon. Sometimes you come across eclectics, who also don't see anything wrong in using finely shredded potatoes in the solyanka – but we will leave such a decision completely up to their conscience. However, pickled mushrooms (especially their flimsy tops!) are highly appropriate and desired in solyanka of every type. Only then can your solyanka turn out to be of the highflying kind – even without slightly salted Atlantic salmon, crawfish necks, or capers. If you don't have pickled mushrooms at home – go down lower on the ladder of possibilities – from fresh to dried, from Boletus to oyster mushrooms, all the way down to marinated ones, but definitely try to find some kind of mushrooms, procure them and put them into the solyanka, otherwise what kind of fish solyanka would it be?!

Don't forget to put a bay leaf into the pot (better into an earthenware pot), crushed fresh black pepper (crushed between two spoons, one inside the other, or with a wide knife, flat side down, on a cutting board), a few grains of fragrant peas, and then, covering the pot with a pot cover, move it for half an hour into a warmed oven or put it on the stove on really low.

Doling out the solyanka into bowls (its thickness should be somewhere on a scale between really rich shchi and regular soup), if you desire it, put a Tbsp of sour cream in each one, sprinkle it with chopped up greens and – this is important! – put in each a triangular piece of lemon, with its skin and seeds removed. There you are! Grab your spoons, as though you're grabbing oars, and row in a friendly way, as though you're on a queen's regatta.

Hash is an entirely different matter. You won't be able to make it in just a few hours or even in an entire day. But there are certain dates on the calendar, when you know beforehand that you'll need the *hash* to restore your organism. *Hash* is an ancient dish, created thousands of years ago with a completely different purpose; there is no doubt that it is older than alcohol. But what does it matter to us when it ideally fits our goal in a given instance. Hash is a kind of flypaper for catching flying alcohol spirits. It's like a police squad that grabs them under their arms and kicks their daredevil company out of the organism no matter how much they want to keep binging. That is why masters of sobering up buy calf or beef legs well in advance, not later than two days before the anticipated festivities.

Speaking roughly, the result should be a hot liquid meat jelly from just cloven-hoofed feet, which, after it has been prepared, is dressed in a special way. But let's take things in good order.

The feet need to be singed and then thoroughly scraped with a knife, washed, and once again scraped, cut up, without harming the bones, and cut at joints and folds (cloven hooves are relatively easy to cut in half along the entire length of the foot with the help of a large sharp knife). In such a partly dissected form they are placed in a large bowl for a day to be rinsed under running water (your conscience will be clean if the thickness of your stream doesn't exceed the thickness of a match, that comprises a flow rate of not more than 40 pails a day, in an extreme case you have to simply change the cold water every two-three hours; in the Caucasus previously they used to wash them, lowering them in a net into a mountain stream). The washed feet are scraped one more time, rubbed, washed – any hints of the burdens of earthly life of large horned livestock are removed – until the bones soften, turn white and acquire the look of well-groomed limbs of creatures, who never trampled the sinful earth.

Then they are cooked for the entire night on the lowest possible setting in a large open pot. The volume of water should evaporate considerably (from 5-6 liters to 1 ½ – calculating for two feet). Only the water and the feet – nothing else, no salt, and no seasonings! This dish, which demands time, requires, however, modest preparation. At the beginning of the boiling process, it is just necessary to skim off a small amount of foam and fat.

When the feet already are boiled soft and begin to fall apart, I, a sinful man, perfectly well understand the "non-canonical nature" of such a decision, but all the same toss into the hash several bay leaves and pepper corns. And I insist that this doesn't ruin the taste of the dish. One should say that the majority of recipes for hash require the presence of boiled tripe among its ingredients, however the work on preparing the tripe is quite labor-intensive, and if you intend to work on it, then it's better to aim at making Polish fliaki (a thick Polish soup made out of tripe), and hash is hash without tripe.

So, you extract the completely soft-boiled feet with a perforated spoon (together with the aforementioned "contraband" spices) and place them on a plate. Allowing them to cool slightly, carefully remove all the bones large and small. What you should have in front of you is a quivering boiled pulp, taken apart by you in small pieces – to get a consistency of something between a jellyfish and a soufflé. By the way, you can suck the bones – in various parts of each one of them there are tiny openings – their juice is quite tasty. If you call your spouse or your children over for help in this endeavor – this undoubtedly will serve to strengthen family bonds. However, let's get to the point.

All the pulp is returned into the bouillon, and you need to bring the hash to a boil. In the meantime on a separate plate you clean and crush no less than a bulb of garlic in a garlic press. Everyone completes the rest on his or her own plate. You can add into the hash only the following ingredients: salt, crushed garlic and vinegar (from half to a full Tbsp of the former and latter – their taste already will be palpable), and additionally, if you so desire, crushed black pepper. Some suggest grated radish instead of vinegar, and also greens and lavash wheat bread to go with the hash. In the end, try it both ways – and make your own judgment. The taste of the hash is red-hot, your lips glue together from it and a warm heaviness sets on the bottom of your stomach, until it occupies all of it in its entirety.

This is the only of the hangover dishes that, by virtue of its specific character and filling nature requires vodka as a necessity, preferably chilled, and possibly – steeped in horseradish (cut the cleaned horshradish root into tiny little cubes and pour it into a half-liter bottle two-fingers high, let it stand several hours). Drink one or three shot glasses (never drink two, because even numbers are seen as bad luck). Take into account that it's best to eat hash during the first half of the day. And take a shower – before and after the hash. This might sound wild and it's nothing but my intuition, but I suspect that alcohol has the tendency to accumulate in the keratinous layers of the epithelium, in the roots of hair and under the fingernails – with these poor relatives of hooves.

What you do after your shower depends on the measure of your preparedness to begin a new (and better) life. To start, I would recommend sleep, as much as you can.

A Holiday from Nothing, or Polish *Bigos*

The tastes of the Slavs, who live at the same geographical latitude, differ among themselves no more than their corresponding Slavic languages. At the basis of this commonality of taste lies a specific heightened acidity, which gives sourness to foodstuff. Pokhlebkin exhaustively spoke about the principle importance of sourness in Slavic cuisines and the truly murderous results of vulgar marinating. That lively sour taste that the Russians so value in their hot *shchi* soups, the Ukrainians – in borscht (especially when it is prepared with beet kvass), the Poles find in their *bigos*. Without a doubt the Polish taste and spirit finds its greatest and fullest expression in this integral dish, which appears as both the first and second hot course simultaneously. The way the sky stands at a distance from the earth, so the *bigos* is distant from that green-sickness, which they love to prepare sometimes more to the south of the Western Bug [pronounced "Boog"] River under the name of "stewed cabbage." The genuine *bigos* is prepared for not less than six hours, but on the other hand you can eat it afterward for a week – on its own, and when you're bored with it – with a side dish of potato puree or fried potatoes. You can even push it into the depths of your refrigerator for an indefinite time, so you can suddenly remember it later. Nothing happens to correctly prepared *bigos*, and it will not lose its taste – despite the fact that culinary authorities write about the undesirability of keeping prepared foods. The notion of *primary* dishes of the three Slavic kitchens – *shchi*, borscht, and *bigos* – in the given case will shame the timid knowledge of the wise.

Thus, bigos (not "bigus," also like "pol'ka" [the accepted pronunciation for a Polish woman] – and not "polyachka" [colloquial pronunciation of the same word]). The main ingredients are: fresh and pickled cabbage. And their ratio depends on your taste, at first try 1:1 (by weight). Take a pot or a deep stewing pan and start to sauté shredded fresh cabbage in a small quantity of heated vegetable oil. The first half hour-hour you'll have to stir it every 5-10 minutes, each time adding just a little bit more vegetable oil. The pot has to be tightly covered. When the cabbage is settled to a third of the original volume and is slightly fried on all sides, continue to do the same thing, each time stirring a handful of the squeezed out (!) pickled cabbage. The cabbage shouldn't burn during the process of being sautéed, but if you start to stew it from the beginning, as a result, whatever you might do, you'll end up precisely with "stewed cabbage."

The kitchen produces a remarkable sense of time in a person. Therefore (while the cabbage is cooking), scrape through every inch of the refrigerator and gather up the maximum amount of varieties of meat products – a little bit of each one: some raw *meat*, preferably of different kinds; *smoked meats* – ring sausages, ham, cooked hot dogs all of a sudden you might find a *kidney* – take everything (you can even take liver and chicken)! *Bigos* is a tornado, sweeping out of the refrigerator all the unutilized scraps, all the leftovers of a festive table. It has been prepared often either on the next day after a lavish party (after the guests something always will be left over), or when among a long train of protracted workdays without a ray of light you felt like organizing a holiday almost out of nothing, in a void, so that life could begin again from the beginning.

You should cut up the meat in cubes, or (if it's firm) beat it with a meat mallet and cut it the way you would for beef Stroganoff. Then fry it on all sides with a large quantity of onions and spices. Under no circumstances salt the meat (otherwise it will release juice) and don't burn it, but just fry it on high until it forms a reddish crunchy crust. Toss the contents of the frying pan into a pot. Also toss into it smoked meat, hot dogs, etc., or whatever else comes to mind, cut up in cubes or shredded. After that add to them a few tablespoons of tomato paste, several scoops of meat bouillon (in the worst case, a bouillon cube dissolved in boiling water – best to use a mushroom-flavored one). Now a very important and obligatory ingredient: a handful of soaked prunes or a few tablespoons of prune preserves (if this is too much for you, then a tablespoon of sugar, though in such a case it would be better and more honest generally to refrain from making bigos, putting off the task for better times).

It will be wonderful if in your household you also find several dried mushrooms (any kind) for the bigos, and if you do, you're one lucky person. The rest is patience. Lower the heat to a minimum under the pot. The bigos will stew itself and the cabbage will release its juice. Once an hour you can visit the kitchen to mix up the contents of the pot with a spoon (this can be either a turkey roasting pan or a regular pan, but they will require more attention, skill, and expenditure of labor and time from you, because they will increase the danger of burning the bigos, which can ruin its taste, which is so rich in nuances).

> *When the thick-brown color of the bigos and an aromatic cloud, shooting up each time from under the slightly raised top, inspire you as quickly as possible to complete the long process of cooking it, do one final thing – add to the bigos no less than 5-6 small bay leaves, two dozen crushed black peppers, a couple of cloves and the same amount of sweet peas), pour in the juice that you strained out of the sauerkraut in the beginning (you don't have to salt the bigos, the sour cabbage has already done this for you), and let it stew for a half hour more on the lowest heat.*

The *bigos* will swim for you in its own juice, the large part of which will be quickly absorbed right after you take off the pot from the heat. Several amateurs add a little more bouillon to the *bigos* at the beginning, so that you can eat it as a thick first course. But intuition suggests that the *bigos* will be even tastier as a juicy second course, with a large quantity of its own aromatic sauce.

One more time:

> –2 pounds of sauerkraut and the same weight (or slightly more) of a fresh head of cabbage;
> –meat, smoked and ringed sausage (various kinds and sorts), from a pound to two;
> –tomato paste, 2-3 Tbsps;
> –prune jam, 2-3 Tbsps or about ten prunes;
> –white or yellow onions, spices;
> –beef bouillon, from 16 to 32 oz;
> –several mushrooms – real good!

In Ukrainian Galicia old women remember how during WWI the scent of ground, black coffee and *bigos* (the Austrian army successfully appropriated the latter) wafted from the Austro-Hungarian trenches in the morning. You can imagine that from the Russian trenches through the rows of barbed wire barriers the odor of kasha wafted over. The morning used to begin gloriously! But no: after fortifying themselves – they began to bludgeon each other with cannons. At this the muse of culinary art falls into silence, together with all the other muses. Especially because a shared meal at a common table at all times, among all nations and civilizations, continues to remain a synonym for peace.

The White Gold of Ukraine

There exist many anecdotes about the heavenly love of Ukrainians for *salo* (pig lard). Here are the reasons for that: *salo*, indeed, occupies a quite exclusive place in the kitchen, and in the national consciousness of Ukrainians. Over the course of hundreds of years it has been a synonym for abundance, stoutness, and profit – a gift of the heavens, the white gold of Ukraine. Gold in so far it is "non-perishable" – in a hot climate all foodstuff spoils quickly, but nothing happens to the salted **salo**. There is nothing easier than salting it, by the way, and it is impossible to oversalt. Rolled into salt it draws in just as much as needed to keep it from spoiling, only 2-3 days are needed for this, the excess of salt then is cleaned off from the *salo's* surface with a knife. If you add hot red pepper to the salt, then you'll end up with so-called "Hungarian *salo*," and if you add crushed black pepper you'll get – "Ukrainian homemade." Ukrainian "migrant workers" always take it with them for the road and to foreign lands and assure that it's impossible to gain weight from it (by the way, the scientific world is of the same opinion regarding *salo* in its pure form). The most delicate taste of the calories of pork *salo*, the bitter sweet crispy antiseptic agents and vitamins of half of an onion, the soft bread acidified by saliva in the accompaniment of a glass of Ukrainian (often homemade) vodka (*horilka*), all of this is of course for a connoisseur, and you have to be healthy to do it.

The harmless attempt anywhere in Germany to prepare an omelet with *salo* or ham will evoke an immediate reaction from the well-bred Germans, with difficulty finding a proper formulation: "Oh, it turns out you have Bavarian taste!" Since long ago they have preferred ground cereals and fruit salads for breakfast, but the familiar odors still stir them, as though they were addicts recovering with difficulty from their addiction. On more than one occasion in West Berlin I happened to catch my landlady with her nose under a pot cover, where Ukrainian borsht was cooking. But that's enough speaking about embarrassing things, even more so, the fact that I don't particularly like finding myself in a railroad car with Ukrainians traveling abroad for work.

Something else is more interesting: why *salo* anyway? William Pokhlebkin in his time pointed out the polemical acuteness of this foodstuff, his evident orientation out of spite or "to spade" (as they say in Ukraine) to their southern neighbors, the Turks and Crimean Tartars. That is, in this way Ukrainians distinguished themselves from them. A pig doesn't like the SOUTH (where it without any basis is considered "unclean"), the NORTH, in as much as it doesn't like cold, and the NOMADIC life, in as much as by nature it is a stay-at-home creature. This settled way of life of the pig, which allows *salo* "to set," is the factor, which, to some degree, "westernizes" Ukrainian cuisine, bringing it closer through Poland and the Czech Republic to the culture of German ring sausages and ham, to Italian *salo* (the best of all) and "marbled" bacon, requiring a refined centuries-old tradition to appreciate it. And the further you go to the East, the less pork you find and the more beef, then mutton and, finally, horsemeat. In Western Ukraine, for example – in Lviv, where I lived for 25 years, the inhabitants of every section of the mid-rise apartment building, even to this day, keep an iron barrel in their basement. Twice a year, right before Christmas and Easter, the barrel is rolled out from the basement into the courtyard, is set up, and everyone in turn cures their meats in it hanging ring sausages, *salo*, *shynka* (ham in Ukrainian), and *shponder* (smoked bacon) – for days and nights on end smoke rises from the courtyards of newly built apartment buildings. The scent of the smoke of fruit tree branches and fresh smoked meats drives both the Uniates and Orthodox crazy, both those who are fasting and those who are not, Roman Catholics, with their shifted Gregorian calendar, and those Jews who've acquired a taste for *salo* (those are mostly the only ones still left in Ukraine), we may say – everyone, including atheists, Hare Krishnas, and business travelers.

Here is the recipe for preparing Galician Ukrainian *shponder* (smoked bacon) at home – essentially this is pork brisket with numerous layers of meat. In other places in Ukraine it's called *podcherevina* (belly bacon), and only in Lviv is it called *shponder* (baked brisket meat), in the German style (simply because the best smoked meats and ring sausages in Galicia even today are made in a particular way in the former German colony of Kulykovo near Lviv where they are made of chopped and not ground meat, and *krovyanka* (bloodwurst) – with buckwheat kasha, and not with *salo* or any other grain, which is made nowhere else in the territory of the former USSR).

Thus, you buy an elongated block of salo with a maximum number of thin vertical layers of meat and with small chopped ribs in the upper part of it. The main law for purchasing meat products is extremely simple: a nice-looking piece, as a rule, turns out to be the tastiest. This kind of piece usually weighs about three pounds. Wash it well with cold water. Then clean a few heads of garlic and, with the help of a sharp narrow knife, insert the garlic cloves into the shponder on all sides and in every direction. Rub the entire piece with salt and slightly with adjika (or pepper it), sprinkle it with dry spices like khmeli-suneli.[48] *In a thoroughly heated roasting pan (or any other kind of pan, but which must be flat-bottomed and made of cast-iron) heat a very small amount of vegetable oil on high (to avoid burning initially) and then fry the entire piece on all sides until a brown tasty crust is formed (not less than 5 minutes for each side). The entire process needs to happen with a tightly closed lid. In the meantime peel several onions and cut them into semicircles. When the shponder is browned on all sides and to the middle, submerged in melted fat, you put the cut up onions into this fat, place the shponder on top of it,*

---

48 *Khmeli-suneli* literally means "dry spices." It is a traditional Georgian spice mix consisting of coriander, dill, basil, bay leaf, marjoram, blue fenugreek, safflower, celery, black pepper, thyme, hyssop, and hot pepper.

> turn down the heat and again cover the roasting pan with a lid. The onions will draw in practically all the fat and with that will become brown and pastose. "Shponder" is a delicacy, a cold hors d'oeuvre; therefore it's eaten cold, with bread. The piquant, well roasted crust; the tender flesh that dissolved the garlic into its body; the onion paste that was fried and stewed at the same time, that absorbed all the juices and aromas, what could be better? You won't need any mustard, sauce or horseradish here! There is one other method: the shponder at first is boiled and then fried in approximately the same way. The taste of boiled shponder is more tender, but weaker.

One piece of advice, concerning *salo* proper: without fail keep it in the freezer. And cut it as thinly as possible, right before using. Then it has a completely ineffable "layered" taste. I understood this some time ago during a long cross-country ski trip on a really frosty day. Later I tested it at home – and it turned out to be true.

Unlike the pig, *salo* loves the cold.

Syr Dariya[49] District Pilaf

There are roughly as many pilafs in the world as there are chefs. Quite a number of Russian people have learned to make it well, having spent some time on different occasions in Central Asia. This recipe was passed along to me by older women, who in the post-war years with hungry eyes used to watch the divine ceremony of Uzbek masters making pilaf. I added a little of my own ad-libbing to it and here is the result.

> You take two pounds of round-grain rice and wash it under running water or let it soak for two hours in salted water.
>
> In a thick-walled cast-iron pot heat no less than 10 ounces of vegetable oil and a bone cleared of meat and a Tbsp of animal fat. It's best of all to have a cauldron for the pilaf, but you can't place it on a modern electric stove, therefore it can

---

49 A district in southern Kazakhstan.

be a roasting pan or even simply a saucepan with a rounded, heavy bottom, which is wider at the bottom. When the bone turns dark, it is thrown out. Place a pound of diced yellow onions into the heated vegetable oil; sauté it for 10 – 15 min while mixing it from time to time, then scoop it onto a plate. Next sauté a pound of carrots, cut them into thin strips or grate them on a grater for Korean carrots, and also scoop them out onto the plate.

Now it's time for 2 pounds of meat. Of course mutton is the classic, but the master of the house is in charge, and I personally prefer chopped pork ribs or even gristle. The meat is seared and braised with zirvak - a mixture of dried barberries, jeera-ajowan-cumin *(all these are various names for Indian caraway) and other spices and flavoring spices, such as* khmeli-suneli, *coriander, Georgian saffron, crushed black pepper, and dried and fresh greens. There should be no less than 50 grams of these spices in dry form. When the meat has been well roasted, but not dried out, it is salted, then flavored with the spices mentioned above, and a glass of boiling water is added to it. The pot is covered with a lid so that the meat can stew with the spices on low heat for about ten minutes. Then the meat is topped with layers of fried onions, carrots, and thoroughly washed rice. If the rice hasn't been soaked in salted water, it's necessary to salt it.*

The rice is slightly sprinkled with turmeric for color with boiling water poured over it, so that it's covered by a ½ inch of water. After about five minutes, when the water steams off and is absorbed by the rice, you stick several cloves of raw garlic into the rice, pat the rice so it becomes thicker and forms a hard surface. You can poke several openings with a round stick so that the moisture evaporates. Do not under any circumstance stir the rice! (By the way, many Eastern peoples consider any kind of boiled crumbly rice a pilaf, and the meat and vegetable part of our pilaf is called zirvak*). Then the pilaf is cooked under the tightly covered lid on low heat for about forty minutes.*

After removing the lid after those forty minutes, you need to check if the rice is ready on the surface – if it's somewhat hard (which is unlikely), you need to make an opening with a little round stick, pour a little boiling water into it and cover the pot with a lid, giving the pilaf another 5-10 minutes before it's ready.

Only then can you mix up the pilaf and lay it out on ceramic plates, which will retain heat longer. Salad made of fresh tomatoes with balsamic vinegar will go amazingly well with it (see the chapter on "Salads. Advice. Recipes").

Beef Liver Pate and Sardines in Tomato Sauce

Nearly everybody loves **liver pate,** but when it is sold in a supermarket or served in a restaurant, it's really easy to fake it. But in just a half hour of actual time you can prepare a pate for canapés for an entire week.

Take 1 ¼ to 1 ¾ pounds of liver (it's better, of course, to use fresh liver) and cut it into pieces about 1/3 to 2/3 inch thick, prick it with a fork and braise it in hot and salted vegetable oil on medium heat. Then in the same frying pan fry about ¾ pound of shredded yellow onions and carrots (you can grate them on a large grater). After letting it cool, chop it all in a food processor, add salt and pepper if necessary, mix a bar of butter into it, place it out in a bowl with a top and put it in the refrigerator. Spread butter and a thick layer of the pate, in which there's not an ounce of extraneous fat, onto a slice of fresh or toasted bread. With a cup of tea this is a ready evening meal or breakfast.

Perhaps not every Russian person loves it, but everyone remembers the taste of sardines in tomato sauce, which is completely unrecognizable in current canned fish products. Having gotten angry and decided that it's not the gods who preserve sardines in tomato sauce,[50] I "invented the bicycle" – and here is the recipe.

---

50 Klekh plays with a Russian saying "It doesn't take gods to make pots" which means

*Take two pounds of any decent type of ocean fish, for example, gray mullet (sufficiently solid so as not to lose its juiciness from possible defrosting on the way to your table, and sufficiently obliging so as to give its juice to the dish). Without defrosting it, clean the scales off it, gut it, chop off the head, wash off the meaty remains and dry it with a paper towel or napkin, chop it into pieces, pepper it, sprinkle it with khmeli-suneli and flour, fry it on a well heated frying pan in salted vegetable oil till a crust is formed, put it in a pot with a bay leaf and at least 3 oz of tomato paste dissolved in 16 oz of boiling water. In the same frying pan sauté one after another about 8 oz of chopped onions, about 10 oz of carrots, shredded or grated on a large grater, and about 1 oz of celery root. Place the sautéed vegetables on top of the fish, add several cloves of black pepper and sweet pea, chopped dry or fresh greens, cover it with a lid, and stew it for about half an hour on low heat. This **fish in tomato** can be kept in the refrigerator and eaten cold, just as those memorable Black Sea sardines, which everyone so enjoyed in his or her childhood in the USSR.*

Let me, perhaps without rhyme or reason, give you a few more pieces of "marine" advice: if you stew squid, know that it is prepared lightning fast, literally in a few minutes, because after 10-15 minutes they harden disastrously, and instead of a tender delicacy, you'll get someone's old shoe sole. Just don't be tempted by fleshy squid that looks so meaty (avoid buying the canned squid too) – these are already nothing but shoe soles. And, for God's sake, never cook already pre-cooked and frozen shrimp (they're red because they've already been cooked), you need to eat them semi-thawed, otherwise they will lose not only their juice, but also the greater part of their taste!

---

that an ordinary man can do complicated things.

Wine and Coffee

Being people of grain and tea, we, all the same, strive to savor the culture of the grape vine and coffee. It's quite amazing that some time ago we had "New Soviet Champagne," Massandra[51] dessert wines, and other things too. It's abominable, that for the great majority of the population, wines, as before, are divided into the "sweet" or "sour" types, and the labels on imported wines are a Chinese puzzle for them. "This is a French wine!" Well, yes, which the bums of Paris drink by the liter on the banks of the Seine because it's cheaper than mineral water. May the experts forgive me, but the rest learn a few of the simplest things. A label on a good wine should be similar to one prepared on an average copy machine – if it's colorful and alluring, they're duping you. Wine for the French is what beer is for the Germans, and vodka – for us. If something bad is happening with vodka, it means something bad is happening in the country. That is why they put you in the slammer in Germany for messing with beer, and in France the winemakers will tear your head off for that sort of businessman – since the time Napoleon III, the despicable usurper, secured the glory of French wine and cognac production (hence Napoleon cognac, with which Bonaparte has nothing to do). It was just then that the winemakers united in guilds, worked out stringent statutes, etc., etc., and began to write honestly on the bottles whether it was table wine, regional, or secured with a code "Appellation control" (that is "require a point of origin control – it would never cross anyone's mind to demand it, the winemakers themselves watch after that, because at this third stage, properly, good wines begin, for which the winemakers answer with their head – and for a long time, and not only in France). By the way, the table wines, and even more so the regional wines also can be superb, but this is simply good luck, an accident; their characteristics are as unstable as those of the Georgian or Moldovan

---

51   The home of Crimea's oldest winery.

wines – they can be amazing for several months, and after a year they turn sour, just like people.

Coffee isn't our forte, though the Turks have long been our neighbors, and we've lived together with the Armenians in one country for a long time. Coffee prepared Eastern style was a sort of a password of the Soviet intelligentsia: it meant "our kind of people"; though back then very few knew how to make it. Now thanks to Italian cafes in large cities, a culture of very fine espresso coffee has taken off, and coffee makers have appeared in stores, which even in the West aren't inexpensive. However, the coffee makers, and the coffee beans, imported wines and exclusive sorts of tea, as should have been expected, are sold in our country for three times the price. As in the anecdote: I buy it for a hundred, sell it for two hundred, and I live on those two per cent. Because this isn't a culture of coffee or wine, but a fad, a social pose of a very fine layer of society. The rest of the people seriously consider instant coffee to be very natural and know all kinds of intricate things about different kinds. This is also a pose, just a slightly more modest one.

You just have to buy coffee beans, but be sure that you roast them (it means nothing that they have already been roasted), finely grind them, and pack them, without sparing, up to a third of the way from the bottom in a *jezve* (or Turkish coffee pot, call it what you like), you can put in some sugar, or make it without, pour boiling water over it, and put it on low heat, mix it and stand over it for several minutes so it doesn't overflow (coffee boiled over is like leftover tea leaves), and leisurely drink strong aromatic coffee from a demitasse coffee cup (and not an American 16 oz mug), smoking a cigarette (caffeine and nicotine neutralize each other, a quarter century ago the journal *Chemistry-Life* wrote about this). There's something to ponder over – something "that wasn't even dreamt by our wise men."[52]

---

[52] From the Russian translation of Shakespeare's *Hamlet*: "There are more things in heaven and earth, Horatio,/ Than are dreamt of in your philosophy."

PART III
Seasonal Culinary Art

A Stitch in Time Saves Nine, or It's Really Helpful to Have a Spoon for Dinner

Only five or six months of the year nourish us, allowing us to fill our organisms with vitamins. Not at any other time of the year vegetables are fruit, berries, and mushrooms, no matter from where they would be brought and how they might be kept, so fresh and revitalizing. From the culinary point of view, the most reasonable and justified course of actions would not be to have a year round "universal greasing" but humbly follow the natural cycles: to make jams in the summer and eat them in the winter, to eat your fill of watermelons and corn in august, to make pickled cabbage in October, to wait for June strawberries, ignoring those that are sold in the supermarket year round, to pick wild raspberries and blackberries, to pickle mushrooms because those produced at factories are insufficiently salted, overcooked, and always tasteless, which is surprising. Even grated German horseradish for some reason is always stronger and purer than our Russian version, which is simply a shame. And let me ask, since when does Russian mustard need preservatives? And if we keep on the subject, where did sushi come from in the middle of the *susha* (dry land) when people living by the sea wait with impatience for the morning catch and for months ending with the letter "R" for fresh fish. And the Moscow gourmets, described by Gilyarovsky, counted the days waiting for the season for fresh oysters?! Alas, all these are just idle questions.

The seasonable nature of eating (like Lent or days of fasting) structures our life and provides a certain kind of unique and inexpensive plot. It is simply NORMAL, while watermelons in January can be seen as a slight psychological abnormality and gastronomic barbarity. Only exotic fruits and vegetables such as pineapples or avocados, which do not grow in our climate and such products as kielbasa and alcohol (with the exception of new vintage wine and freshly brewed beer) can be consumed year round, and everything that grows in a given climate zone and in nearby neighboring countries is better to consume during the proper season, welcoming and parting with products in turn. Of course, it is conservatism, but it is a healthy conservatism and its absence results in turning all products into food garbage without exception. It is stupid to break into an opened door, but what can you do when civilization deliberately strives for the elimination of seasonal changes, to independence from weather, the climate, and the aureole of habitation, toward turning the entire world into artificial honeycombs of little homogeneous synthetic worlds? Isn't it time to try at least to slow down this process?

The Modest Beauty of the Lenten Table

Lent is not a diet (that is, a culinary sectarianism when people do it out of idleness or curiosity), but an experiment in suppression of lust in the broadest sense of the word. It is not up to me to expound on the religious motives of Lent, but at one time in my youth, I was shamed by my acquaintance, who said to me: "Could you at least not eat meat on Good Friday?" She wasn't a very strong believer but respected traditions and continued observing the rituals. On Christmas Eve and for Easter she and her husband invariably invited friends – Russians, Ukrainians, and Jews to their house and treated them with a holiday dinner. It is in their home I forever became absorbed by the indisputable beauty of the Lenten table, which I would like to share with my readers now.

Christmas Eve, called Bountiful Evening awakens in people the memory of their childhood when the presence of the Christmas tree moved the walls apart, exciting the senses and promising New Year miracles and amazing presents. Adults are always a little sad on that day. Because of the discrepancy between the Soviet and church calendars, our New Year preceded our Christmas, which disrupted the logic of holiday feasting. For the New Year we eat and drink indiscriminately in large quantities, but the festive table on Christmas Eve is quiet and austere, being an expectation of the momentous holiday and, because of that, flickers and shines with symbols – from the life and death of the wheat grain in the *kutya* (the thick wheat gruel served for remembering the souls of the deceased) to baked or jellied fish as an ideogram and the code of Jesus Christ (Ichthys – IHS). Ideally on that day there should be twelve dishes on the table. The first, most archaic and complex because of its simplicity, is **kutya**. However, there are very few people who are familiar with authentic *kutya*, which demands the highest culinary skills for its preparation and does not allow the substitution of Asian rice for the Slavic grain.

The best kutya of those that I have tasted is prepared in the following way. Boil 1 cup of wheat in 2 cups of water for 3 hours. Meanwhile pour a cup of boiling water over a cup of poppy seeds. When the water cools down, drain it and grind the poppy seeds with a mortar and pestle for 40 minutes until the poppy seeds become lumpy. Add a cup of sugar to the ground poppy seeds and continue grinding until the sugar is completely absorbed by the mixture. Right before serving the kutya, mix the wheat broth and the whey with ground poppy seeds and add 1 tablespoon of honey (although some people prefer unsweetened kutya, which is quite appropriate at wakes). When the ingredients are not mixed together, the kutya can be kept in a refrigerator for several days without any detrimental effect to its taste.

For the first course you should serve **borsht with "ears"** *– tiny pelmeni (dumplings) stuffed with boiled mushrooms (the mushrooms can also be sautéed with onions). The distinct feature of this borsht is that it is cooked for quite a long time without cabbage and tomatoes, and when it is ready, all the vegetables are removed and only the "ears" are left in the broth.*

Fresh water carp (up to 2 lbs.) is ideal for making aspic (the only thing you have to do is to remove the thin forked bones that go along the spine).

To increase the number of dishes, you can bake small cabbage pies, prepare Lenten salads out of grated radishes or cooked beans with onions and crushed garlic – which is not difficult, tasty beyond belief and refreshing. Desert can only be one thing – the compote "Uzvar" (which can be called the Ukrainian national drink for Christmas Eve) made out of dried fruits with the predominance of small pears in the mixture. It is such a great drink and chaser.

Even an incorrigible atheist and drunkard, after seeing the first star on Christmas Eve, can be tamed and become better by experiencing such a bountiful table in contrast to how he looked indulging in the noisy New Year Eve festivities or stupidly surfing channels on the TV.

Kholodets (cold jellied meat) is not *studen* (cold gelatin meat)

The main difference between the South Russian and Ukrainian **kholodets** (cold jellied meat) and the Northern *studen* (cold gelatin meat) is in the fact that pig's feet are used for preparing *kholodets* and beef and veal – for *studen*. In older days *studen* became a cold dish when a cattle head was boiled for it, but who can do such a terrible thing today? It is customary for Russians to boil beef to the point that the meat comes apart, to add a lot of gelatin and call the dish *studen'*. Pig's feet skin, or fore shanks, hooves, and cartilage discharge a jellying substance on their own, and this gives the dish unmatched taste. *Kholodets* uses not only the meat of pig's feet but also hard-boiled beef or chicken, and because of this the dish is optimal for the cold table. Here's how you cook it.

It is better to use the pig's feet "with boot tops" (they have more skin and stringy hog-chocks inside). Carefully scrape and soak them in water for a little while. Scour the skin on all joints and bends and cook them uncovered in a large pot on low heat, adding 1 onion, 1 carrot, 1 small parsley root, bay leaf, and a whole pepper to the pot (you will discard all the vegetables and spices after you are done). Bring it to a boil, skimming the mixture until clear. Reduce heat and simmer for 5 hours, until the time when the pig legs start to break at the joints. 2 hours before that add a piece of beef, veal, or chicken and 1 fresh carrot to the mixture. A film of fat will inevitably form on the surface of the broth. Skim it off so it doesn't spoil the appearance of the kholodets when it cools down and jells. After the bones come apart and approximately two thirds of the water evaporates, take the meat out, separate it from the bones (you may want to suck juice from the pork bones through the tiny holes – you may find them very tasty), discard all vegetables and spices except for the second carrot. Generously salt the broth, add 4 -5 cloves of crushed garlic and 1 – 2 Tbsp of vinegar. Sift the broth through a cheesecloth and return it to a cleaned saucepan. Taste the broth – it has to have a robust taste because when the kholodets is ready, the harshness will be gone and the taste will be mellow. Dissolve a packet of gelatin in water according to the packet instructions (without the gelatin the kholodets will jell but it will melt when you put it on the table). When the gelatin expands, add it to the broth, mix it well, and simmer for a while without bringing the broth to a boil. Cut the beef into thin slices and place all meats with the skin side up into a serving dish for the kholodets (it could be a shallow bowl or a casserole dish with a lid), decorate with carrot slices (you may also use slices of a hardboiled egg if that works for you), lemon triangles, and parsley and celery leaves. All that is left is to carefully pour the broth (watch out and don't spoil the beauty of the arrangement) over the meat and let it cool before transferring it to the refrigerator. The ideal condiment for the kholodets is **grated horseradish with beets** (cook the beets, add lemon juice, salt, sugar, ground black pepper to your liking), strong mustard or mustard diluted with vinegar, and the **black radish salad** with sunflower oil (don't forget to salt the radish and squeeze the juice out of it, so that you don't get heartburn).

Pelmeni (meat ravioli) are not *Varenyky* (cottage cheese or cherry dumplings)

Pelmeni are considered to be a dish from the Perm area that came to Siberia from China, and because it has been appropriated by the

Russian kitchen for many centuries, it received the name Siberian *pelmeni*. In Siberian villages the *pelmeni* were made by the entire family; they were taken outside to freeze, and bags of them were made every winter. This is the first unique aspect of the Siberian *pelmeni*: they are better tasting and cook better if you freeze them. The second unique feature consists of the "non-Russian" *meat stuffing*: at a minimum it is a mixture of ground beef and pork, which becomes especially piquant if you add a little bit of ground lamb or horsemeat and, in addition, finely cut or grated onion, a little bit of garlic or buckram, dill, parsley, salt, black pepper, raw egg, and a couple of tablespoons of beef broth.

For those who love numbers: 1 lb. of ground beef + ¾ lb. of ground pork + ½ lb. of ground lamb or horsemeat, 5 oz. of onion, 1 oz. of crushed garlic, 1 oz. of dill and parsley, less than 1 Tbsp. of salt, and pepper to taste. Finally, we come to the dough. Some believe that it is supposed to be very thin and very stiff in order not to make it difficult for the stomach to digest the boiled dough and to prevent the stuffing from falling out of the pelmeni. But when you roll out the stiff dough for a while, your hands will hurt for a couple of days. There is another simpler and more effective method to kill two birds with one stone: don't make the dough with iced water but with sour cream – this kind of dough will not stick in your teeth or become a brick in your stomach, and it doesn't have to be rolled as thin as possible. Use 2 lbs. of sifted flour, 1 cup of sour cream, 1 Tbsp. of salt, 2 Tbsp. of sugar, and 2 eggs. Knead the dough with both hands to a proper consistency, pounding it on the table; if it feels too stiff, add cold milk diluted with water, if you think the dough is too soft, add more flour. When you feel working with the dough becomes easy, roll it into a ball, cover it with a kitchen towel, and let it stand for a while so that it acquires a uniform consistency. It is sadistic to suggest that you make pelmeni by hand – use a pelmeni (or ravioli) maker. Dust the lower sheet with flour, place the thinly rolled (1 – 2 mm) sheet of dough on it, and slightly depress it into the openings (the elastic, sour cream-based dough stretches much better than a stiff one), put the balls of ground meat into these indentations with a wet spoon, sprinkle a similar sheet of dough with water and place it on the ravioli maker with the moistened side down, press the lumps of the stuffing down and roll the pin over the dough to make the ridge separating the pelmeni. Put a dusting of flour on the ravioli maker, turn it over, and knock on it to dump out the pelmeni. Place them on the flour-dusted board or dish and then put it in the freezer (in half an hour to an hour you can put them in a freezer bag to store or cook them). To prevent them from being overly crowded, you should cook the pelmeni in a large, wide pot with a large quantity of boiling salted water. You should drop them into the rapidly boiling water, carefully stirring them with a wooden spoon, skimmer, or spatula with a long handle. The water temperature drops sharply when you put the pelmeni in. That's why it is so important to catch the moment when the pelmeni start to rise to the surface and the boiling resumes. As they do that, you should reduce the heat, and in the worst case, even turn it off adding cold water to the pot as you extinguish the coals under the grilled shishkebab. You should boil pelmeni for about 10-15 min after they come to the surface, and the water should boil in a way that the pelmeni don't crowd each other or turn somersaults, but lazily stir in the boiling water. Pelmeni cooked in concentrated spiced beef broth are very tasty, as is customary with the Turkic peoples. When made this way the pelmeni are eaten in the bouillon like a soup, sprinkled with pepper and greens. But even if you decide to cook the pelmeni in the water that you will later pour out, when you drain the pelmeni in a colander, treat that water as a type of broth: don't begrudge using a cross-cut onion, bay leaf, and a few crushed peppercorns in it. You can even oversalt the broth, pelmeni will just thank you for that. Let the water drain for about 30 sec. After that put the pelmeni into a porcelain bowl with melted butter, and covering it with a lid, shake it a few times. Serve the pelmeni right after that with warmed up sour cream, pepper, soy sauce, whatever you love. There are people who like to leave a few pelmeni for the next day, frying them covered with salo or mayonnaise so that they won't dry out.

Damn, this makes my mouth water. I'm going for a shot of vodka. I'll be right back after that.

For their varenyky (cottage cheese or cherry dumplings), which they borrowed from the Turks, the Ukrainians use the same trick as the Russians for their sour cream-based dough for the pelmeni, the only difference is that they use cottage cheese for their celebrated "cheese pyrohy" which might kill you because it's impossible to stop eating them. Once when I was in the Poltava region in Ukraine, I wondered: where is the dough in the varenyky? Is it thinner than paper if I don't feel it? It turned out that it is just the opposite: when it is boiled soft, the dough becomes several times thicker than pelmeni dough, but it does not feel heavy because it has the tender consistency of the so-called "lazy varenyky." In combination with natural farmer-made sour cream, it is an absolutely killer dish that is quite easy to prepare in today's Russia. Cottage cheese is best suited for the stuffing: take 1 lb. of cottage cheese, 1 egg, and ½ Tbsp. of sugar, mix all the ingredients and knead. To make the dough, take 1¼ lb. of flour, 5 oz. of cottage cheese, 4 oz. of milk, 2 Tbsp. of sour cream, 1 egg, ½ Tbsp. of sugar, and ½ Tbsp. of salt. Knead the dough and let it stay covered until it settles. Don't make varenyky using circles, by cutting out the rolled dough with the rim of a glass, because you'll waste a lot of dough this way. It's better to use the same technique as when you make Russian mini-pies (pirozhki), that is by rolling the dough into a small log, cutting it into small pieces, shaping each piece into a disk with your hands, and flattening them to a thickness of a tenth of an inch." Put the stuffing on them, wet the edge with cold water, and carefully pinch the varenyk in the shape of a half-moon. Cook the varenyky just like the pelmeni in a large, wide pot, filled with mildly boiling water for 10-15 min. The cooked varenyky also like butter and thick sour cream, and they cool down very quickly – don't let them do that.

Two more types of varenyky need to be mentioned. First of all, it is varenyky **with berries***, and above all with cherries. The trick here is to dry out the berries a little bit so that the varenyky do not fall apart in the boiling water. To achieve this, cover the pitted cherries (or plums) with sugar, and let them sit for a couple hours. After that, decant the juice to the last drop and use it for making sugar syrup, which will be used for the cooked varenyky – it is smart and economical. You can also use the juice for something else and eat the varenyky with sour cream and sugar, but you should cook them in lightly salted water. Another bit of varenyky know-how with Russian/Ukrainian variations is varenyky with mashed potatoes (that is, a variation of the Polish pierogies), which have been boiled unpeeled. In the Russian kitchen the stuffing includes sautéed onions and mushrooms. In the Ukrainian kitchen – "shkvarky" (pork rinds), pieces of pig lard are fried with onions, which either are included in the stuffing or used as a hot sauce for the varenyky. You cannot allow varenyky to go cold, but you can prepare them in advance and keep them in the freezer until it is time to use them. They will lose something in the process, but also gain some new qualities.*

In Nikolai Gogol's story "Old World Landowners" from his celebrated collection of stories from Ukrainian life *Mirgorod* (1835), the character Afanasy asks his neighbor: "Shouldn't we, esteemed Pulkheria Ivanovna, eat some *varenyky* with cherries in such accursed weather?"

"Why shouldn't we," she answers.

Let's follow their suggestion.

Kasha, Porridges, and Gruels

Hot cereals are divided into three kinds – hard kasha, gruel, and porridge (soup-like porridge). In our childhood, it would seem, we all ate nothing but gruels. Even now I shudder when I think of the thickly made semolina or rice porridge with jam spread on top. That is why I am not going to discuss porridges at all.

The super cool king of hot cereals is undoubtedly buckwheat kasha. There is nothing easier to cook than it. It doesn't come out right for many people or doesn't work out at all just as a result of laziness. First, the buckwheat has to be select, but even this kind has to be carefully sorted out, for which you should spread it on the table and then dry and lightly brown it on a frying pan or baking sheet at a temperature of 200 – 300° F. Second, the lightly salted buckwheat is covered with boiling water – 2 cups for 1 cup of grain and boiled with a cover on for 4 mins on high, 4 mins on medium, and 4 mins on low. After you see that the water has been absorbed by the kasha, add butter without holding back. This is something you should memorize like the multiplication table or rules of grammar – the water to grain proportion is 2:1 and the saying "you can't spoil your kasha with butter" (which is very true for all hard kashas and porridges). Finally, something that even diligent people often neglect to do, the kasha should still reach its right consistency by stewing in a warm oven for at least half an hour. We prefer to wrap the saucepan filled with the kasha in a towel, while all we have to do is make the decision to find and buy a clay pot (or several small ones that can also be used for cooking meat stew with potatoes or chanakhi, stewed lamb with vegetables, or whatever you want). If you just cook the kasha one time in the right way, you will understand how much we lose as a result of our own laziness. The kasha is as magnificent by itself and also as a side to meat stew, or simply flavored by sautéed onions.

In order to cook **non-sticky rice**, *the proportion of water and rice should be 1 ½ - 1. The sorted out, non-steamed, long-grain rice is rinsed under cold water for 10 mins to remove the rice flour. After that, the rice is poured into hot salted water and cooked with bay leaf added until all the water is completely absorbed. Then the rice is sprinkled with vegetable oil, or butter* *is spread on it and kept covered for a few minutes with the heat turned off; it is better if this is done not in the saucepan, but in a cauldron or clay pot (if the rice is not cooked on an open fire).*

Gruels *are a different matter. Even the semolina kasha, which I have hated since childhood because it always stuck like a lump in my throat, if it is cooked in milk like a thin soup (1 Tbsp. is added to 1 cup of slightly salted hot milk and cooked while being stirred on low heat for about 10 mins) can light up your morning with the hope for a quiet and successful day. The same can be said about pumpkin milk gruel, which smells so intoxicatingly with pumpkin seeds (but the pumpkin pulp first has to be minced and cooked in a small amount of water until it is completely soft).*

Sweets and Whims

Only in passing do we touch on tea pastries, because dilettantes have no place in a pastry bakery, this most elite area of culinary art. But I do not even claim expertise. All I want is to have something cooked in a hurry for tea.

First, let's talk about whims – dry **caraway seed pastry***. Sift 3 cups of flour, add 2 sticks of softened butter or margarine, 2 eggs, 1 cup of warm milk, 1 ½ tsp of salt, 1 ½ tsp of sugar, and 1 oz. of caraway seeds (you can substitute for it with the same amount of sesame seeds or ¼ lb. of grated cheese). Knead the dough and flatten it to a thickness of 0.1". Cut the sheet into circles with a wine glass and place them on a buttered baking sheet (pinprick the pastries with a fork so that the dough won't puff up). Place the baking sheet in an oven pre-warmed to 360°F. In about 20 mins start watching the pastries so that the browning does not turn into burning (the pastry is very thin and can burn in 5 mins). If you do that, in no more than a half an hour you will have a plate full of such aromatic, crunchy, dry crackers that you can't buy anywhere.*

You can also bake short prianiki (gingerbread or spice cakes), which, even when they dry, will not go stale for weeks. The secret is in the amount of fat that goes in it. For 1 ½ lbs. of flour use 6 oz. of sugar, 6 oz. of butter, margarine or lard (don't be shocked, try it), 2 oz. of sour cream, 1 Tbsp. of vegetable oil, 1 egg, 1 tsp of baking soda, 1 tsp of vanilla extract, a splash of lemon juice, a pinch of ginger or another natural aromatic spice like cardamom, and a ½ shot glass of cognac or strong liqueur (a sacred ingredient in baking). Form balls 1½ – 2" in diameter and place them on a baking sheet 1½-2" apart (baked at 400 °F, the balls will settle down and take the shape of flat prianiki). It goes without saying that the pastry should be placed in a pre-heated oven.

People of my generation will never forget our mothers' Napoleons prepared with custard, but I doubt that children of other generations will be able to appreciate the beauty of this torte of impoverished days. Nevertheless it would be cruel to leave a modern mother without a recipe for some fairly simple cake for a family holiday, such as **plum or prune cake.**

Dough is made by combining 1 lb. of seethed flour, 1 cup of sugar, 3½ oz. of honey, 3½ oz. of sour cream, 2 whisked eggs, 1½ tsp of baking soda, a dash of salt, and 1 oz. of cognac or strong liquor. Carefully knead the dough and let it cool down in the refrigerator for an hour. Divide the dough into three parts and bake in a round baking dish with the removable side (each layer is baked for 20 min at 400 °F). Cool down the layers, cut off any bulges and crush them (the crumbs will be used for sprinkling on top of the cake). For making the filling, pour boiling water over 1 lb. of prunes and cook for 5 mins. Cool the prunes down and finely cut. Crumble ¾ lb. of butter and mix with 1 Tbsp. of sweet condensed milk. Add the prunes and spread the mixture over the cake layers. Sprinkle the top layer with the cake crumbs and/or crushed nuts and put the cake into the refrigerator to cool for 6 to 10 hours where it will become richer.

> We won't stoop as low as to offer a recipe of the "charlotte" (a Russian apple pie), but there is nothing easier to prepare than a **baked apple** for desert. Cut out the core of a sour-sweet apple, pour 1 tsp of sugar or honey in the cutout, cover it with the cut out cone with the stalk, cover the apple with 2 layers of aluminum foil, and put it in the oven to soften it. You will end up with a portion of a wonderful apple soufflé. Take a teaspoon and dig in to the sweet delicacy.

The Desire for Soup

"On the evening of January 11 the huge auditorium of The Hermitage Museum would be transformed. The expensive, silk-upholstered furniture would disappear, the floor would be thickly covered with sawdust, and simple wooden tables, stools, and Viennese chairs would be brought in…. Only cold dishes, vodka, beer, and cheap wine would be left in the buffet and kitchen. It was the people's holiday in the bourgeois palace of gluttony.…" That is how Gilyarovsky described the traditional student feast on Tatiana's Day (the day of the great martyr Tatiana of Rome, which also was the day commemorating the opening of Moscow University and thus a holiday for students) at famous chef Messier Olivier's establishment. It looks very picturesque and even inspired you if you were young and constantly hungry. I remember how greedily during the decline of the Soviet epoch we jumped at all those stand-up receptions, buffets, and smorgasbords at various presentations and gatherings: "Freebies, ladies and gentlemen!" Notwithstanding the fact that the "freebie" was a drug, many have managed to smother their appetite since that time.

The stand-up receptions with cold dishes (even those that include hot dishes such as shish kebabs or the unfortunate julienne) are nothing more than a cold food table. I am no longer warmed up by its offerings or by chaotic corporate get-togethers. In the last two decades they were necessary for something – for preserving the caste structure or simply for preventing people from turning sour in shameless loneliness (even negative sensations can be the food for your soul of which Kafka said it best in his diaries: "How refreshed you feel after a conversation with a blithering fool."). However, I think that nowadays their time is coming to an end and the sphere of their usefulness has narrowed. It is still wonderful to drink a glass of chilled white wine or ice-cold vodka, chasing it with a piece of cheese or a pickle or a pickled herring canapé at an art opening or literary presentation – but not to jostle around among art works, books, and acquaintances with a plate in your hand, which is chaotically heaped with all kinds of stuff for future use. What is more, the better the dishes, the worse the result of their mindless proximity in your stomach. Enough! The hosts and organizers of the receptions should not provoke their guests or corrupt their employees with unprincipled freebies.

I feel like eating hot soup. You'll say it is a sign of approaching old age, but I've wanted to eat it for long time and virtually every day. In my childhood I didn't want it at all. The first time I felt like I wanted hot soup was when I was around 30 and had divorced my first wife. A few months after the divorce, I suddenly felt that I was acutely missing something. After I gave it a good think, it dawned on me: I wanted soup!

I had to cook it myself, and until now its vivid image stands in front of me. Vapors rise above the side of the bowl where sour cream shows white, sparkles of oil – yellow, and eyelashes of dill – green; and where finely cut potatoes and close-grained stalks of cauliflower rest on the bottom. A spoon is in one hand, a slice of bread in the other, and your mouth waters like crazy. Also – two friends at the table who only then began to realize the great role of soup in the life of a Russian person.

Nowadays the simplest soup can be easily improved upon by making it a **three-cabbage soup** *– using white or savoy cabbage (which is beautiful but not very juicy), cauliflower, and broccoli (and if you partially substitute potatoes with sliced or cubed kohlrabi (turnip-cabbage, it will become a four-cabbage soup). Every 5 mins put the kohlrabi, potatoes, bay leaf, cauliflower,* *and finally white cabbage and dill and parsley roots and stalks lightly sautéed in the heated and salted vegetable oil into the boiling vegetable broth. Turn the heat off, add salt to the taste, add 1 Tbsp. of butter, and let it stand covered for 5 mins. All that is left is to pour the soup into the bowls, add sour cream, sprinkle it with greens, pepper it, and take the spoons. The entire cooking process including preparation takes about half an hour, but it will make you happy for at least half of a day.*

The Formula for Borsht

As there are rain people, so there are borsht people. One of my good friends, a native of Russia, frowned at any feeble impulse to cook something other than borsht as the first course and after a few moments asked: "What do we not have to make borsht?" There is something pan-Slavic in this dish. Borsht is a metaphor for summer, for which every Slav waits and longs. That is why borsht has to be served not just hot, but scorching hot, scorching with the afternoon summer heat. Even its name is glorious – borsht! It sticks to your ear like a bur, like a password. No doubt that it is an integrated dish, and many versions of it exist – Moscow, Polish, etc. However, the full intensity, the full expression of its qualities, its quintessence is reached more to the South, in Ukraine with its baroque taste and excessive fleshiness.

In Moscow restaurants, the borsht is cooked by famous foreign chefs as a culinary "hit" – they have the full right to do so, but let's find the courage to present its Ukrainian and also South Russian versions in the way in which it exists today. The kitchen is the same battlefield as the entire field of culture, with its own schools, heresies, deviations, and expansions. It is quite possible that a kitchen history of civilization will be written one of these days. Nevertheless, blood, and not human blood after all, is present there only in blood sausage and English roast beef.

Of course, we can recall how during the Russian Civil War of 1918-1921, the leader of the Ukrainian anarchist army, Nestor

Makhno, hanged the plant-selection breeder Lev Simirenko (supposedly the inventor of the Simirenko Reinette apple) for the latter's infringement on the prerogative of the Creator or how Muslims are "driven bonkers" by pig's ears. But enough of an introduction, let's move closer to the matter at hand!

The culinary art is one of the forms of the applied arts, and a chef is always partly an artist because he *a priori* possesses an aesthetic image and concept of the dish he is preparing. When you begin cooking, you must imagine how you are going to bring forward the taste of the original product or components of the future dish, what you need to extinguish and neutralize in it, what – to intensify, what should be the progression of your actions in order that the result be harmonious. But the result is always unique because you deal not with simple chemical elements, but (until very recently) live organisms. To cook, to boil means to revive the, alas, already not living matter, to nurture a taste that is filled with living power.

Thus the borsht about which the author is preaching and the concepts of which he upholds here must be:

Hot, even scorching, as mentioned above, although during one of the subsequent mornings it's good to slurp down its cold broth, which is, without a doubt, the tastiest component of a successfully cooked borsht. In this extract, in this liquid, as in a magnifying glass, all the taste components of borsht are focused. For someone it would seem crazy to keep the borsht standing for a day or even several days, because everyone remembers the maxim about one-day cabbage soup. However, properly cooked borsht is not susceptible to growing old, one can even say it is imperishable and is steeped in the refrigerator in the same way as it is on a stove. Even more so because its cooking is labor-effective with regard to time (1 ½ – 2 hours), and it must be cooked in a large pot, not less than 2 ½ – 3 quarts capacity. However, the author of these pages admits that his tastes in this question are the most plebeian and democratic.

Of course the borsht should be **rich**. *What does this mean? First, cook the broth: use a good bone (it is better if it is a marrow* bone with meat) and a lot of filtered water (remember that one third of water will evaporate during cooking). The broth is made by simmering the bone in a large uncovered pot for 2 to 4 hours. It is cooked with almost no participation on your side. All you have to do is to wash and put the meat into the water, skim it a couple of times, add herbs and vegetables – an onion, carrot, and parsley root (you may want to bake the onion beforehand and replace the parsley root with a turnip, but some white root is absolutely necessary – there can be no doubt about it). You also put a bay leaf and 10 black peppercorns in the broth. As a result we will have the yet unsalted meat broth strained through a cheesecloth or a fine strainer and the deboned boiled meat on a platter. The rest is discarded.

The taste of the cooked borsht should be:

a. sour-

b. sweet-

c. spicy-hot.

Tomato paste and sour cream (added into the bowl of borsht) will make it sour. If you feel that the tomato paste or its sourness is not enough to make the borsht sufficiently sour, boldly add 1 Tbsp. of vinegar or lemon juice to the soup – any means are good in the culinary arts to achieve your goal. The use of tomatoes in addition to the tomato paste will make the taste of the borsht more airy, more summer-like, and less concentrated. The same goal can be achieved by adding sweet green or red peppers, sliced into circles, although such solutions will take us away from the basic, orthodox formula for borsht. Borsht's sweetness is achieved primarily by the use of carrots, but if you feel that is not enough, courageously add a tsp of sugar.

Finally, the spiciness. Its main ingredient is red chili pepper, ten or so ground black peppercorns and several kernels of clove, and finally – right before you turn the borsht off – garlic crushed with sea salt and frozen salo (you may chop and grind everything with a wide knife, if you want to get a real Ukrainian borsht, no kidding).

Finally, the borsht must be an extremely **red color** *(don't begrudge the beets and tomatoes), with a sparkling surface, and yellow scales of fat spots. We will* **make it white** *in bowls by adding the sour cream and enliven it with thinly chopped greens (mainly dill).*

That is the foundation of it.

But we should not omit several important details. Approximately a half an hour before the borsht is ready, sauté the thinly chopped onions, carrots, parsley root, along with the dill and parsley stems in the vegetable oil, in a deep frying pan. Add grated beets; sprinkle it with vinegar or lemon juice and sauté the mixture for another 5 – 10 mins. Clear a space on the frying pan and add a Tbsp. of flour (it will later impart the broth with the desired "thickness" and barely discernable "meatiness"), mix everything once again, add a half cup of tomato paste (the Iranian or Mediterranean would be the best because it has no additives – just tomatoes, water and salt, with 25% consistency), a couple of ladles of broth, cover and sauté it until the beets are almost soft. It would be a good idea to use a pinch of a mixture of dried spices – hop sprouts (Georgian [from the Caucasus region] are better than the Polish ones).

Meanwhile, add cubed potatoes (nowadays potatoes are cooked for about 20 min) to the strained and lightly salted broth.

Not sooner than 10 min before you turn the heat off (depending on the season), add shredded white cabbage to the broth (by the way, if you cook it very early in the summer, don't miss out on using the young beets with tops because the beet tops will replace the cabbage and make the taste of the borsht closer to beet-root soup – this kind of "youthful" borsht you can eat only one month of the year).

It is very important not to overcook the vegetables; the sense of freshness of the borsht will depend on this. In a couple of minutes after you've added the vegetables, add the contents of the frying pan to the pot, plus a bay leaf, half of a hot chili pepper, and other spices. The above-mentioned garlic ground with salt and salo is added last immediately before turning the heat off (you do not have to do it, if it turns you off, but without it you will lose an important component of the Ukrainian borsht).

Next comes the taste sampling, the elimination of extremes, and making the last corrections. The borsht should be left standing slightly under-salted and under-peppered on the turned-off stove, covered with a towel over the lid. The borsht should spend up to a half hour standing on a heated stove. During that time, left to itself, it will draw from its components what they did not yield during the cooking process, will appease the pot's passions, and harmonize the mutual claims of its components.

Don't forget about thinly chopped dill and fresh sour cream (which, alas, you cannot find in many countries nowadays). In the world of dairy products, it occupies the same place as Russia in the world of geography. It is not the Protestant sour top milk, or the curdled milk of the steppe nomads, or the *matzoon* (fermented milk) of the mountain people; it is the butter of the lazy and possesses that tender consistency and characteristic sourness, which are so near and dear to the Slavic stomach. If you are not a teatotaler, it would be very much advisable to precede your eating of the borsht with a shot of chilled vodka.

It goes without saying that you should never eat the borsht alone.

"*Smachnoho!*" (Bon appetite! – as they say in Ukrainian)

It is not desirable to overlook any one of the ingredients in the borsht. It would be the equivalent of missing a note or a beat in a culinary composition, or, what might be even worse, a mistake in a recipe.

It goes without saying that what was stated above is just an outline, a musical score, or a generalized image, because there is no single kind of borsht. There are different kinds of borsht – an entire class of first courses, crawling out in all directions like crayfish dumped out onto a road. Even if we limit ourselves to just the Ukrainian borsht, we are flabbergasted.

Each province desires to have its own borsht – Kyivan, Chernihovan, Volynian, there is no end to them. And while the people of Poltava use the sugar beet instead of the red beet and add sliced cucumber to it, people in Kremenchuk may offer you borsht… without beets at all. "We never put *buryaky* (beets) in borsht!" They say with dignity to a dumbfounded traveler, although borsht is in fact the beet, the *buryak*, and Dalwrote about it a hundred and fifty years ago: "Borsht is pickled beets; a kind of cabbage soup, made out of pickled beets with a base of beef or pork broth.…" In Soviet times there was even a railroad capitol of borsht – Romodan in Western Ukraine where the train stopped for not less than twenty minutes so that the passengers could try the hot borsht right there under canopies on the platform and, thus strengthening themselves, continue their journey. The train schedules were adjusted accordingly.

At some places you can be offered borsht based on chicken bouillon – a clear sign of the close proximity to the Jewish settlements in the times of old, or in Western Ukraine – a borsht with ham and hot dogs (which is called in the culinary books either "Lviv borsht" or "sailors' borsht," or even "Moscow borsht") – a dish marked by the Uniate[53] spirit that came into existence, most likely, under pressure of the Polish *bigos* and German tastes.

There are attempts to impart to borsht a universal character by introducing prunes and other dried fruits or fermented bread juice, making the borsht the first, second, and third courses at the same time, a kind of *prix fixe* dinner – you eat just borsht and you are filled.

Borsht can be embellished only with mushrooms, and/or kidney or pinto beans. It will also not be spoiled by *halushkas* (Ukrainian dumplings), sauerkraut with pickled apples, and even lamb (only no kind of fish should be used in the borsht, though I have some fiends who like that). Like a living creature or melting pot, the

---

53 The Uniate church was introduced at the Union of Brest in 1596 to allow the Byzantine church in Ukraine to be in union with the Roman Catholic Church.

insatiable borsht is ready to absorb ("*zasmoktaty*" in Ukrainian) and digest everything. Let's say it this way: all variations of borsht and its relatives may come out tasty and appetizing if you manage to feel its ideological paradigm orientation and the basic sensory motif of this dish, which I have tried to deconstruct and then put back together here as a *formula for borsht*.

Borsht teaches people one extremely important lesson that goes far beyond the limits of the culinary art – it teaches us as the Russian language itself prompts us – not to over-*borsht-it* (*pereborshchivat'*) [to go over the top].

Maslenitsa (Shrovetide),[54] *Blin!*[55]

What is left for us from the Shrovetide festivities is just *bliny* and Forgiveness Sunday, which maybe is not that bad. No longer do we need to ride the Russian hills ("to ride the hills, to wallow in *bliny*"), or hold dashing fistfights, or the necessary fraternizing with mothers-in-law, or the rather horrifying rite of the Kostroma burning.[56] But the *blin*, being a solar sign and hand-made imprint of celestial bodies and resembling the lunar landscape with its blistered surface, is archaic in the extreme. By the way, has it ever crossed your mind that our tea drinking from a *samovar*, cups, and saucers[57] very closely resembles our solar system? Food is food, but kitchen is a theater of ideological spectacles. *Maslenichnaya* (the adjectival form of Shrovetide, from the word "*maslo*" [that which is being spread]) or Cheesefare Week (when in anticipation of the

---

54   Maslenitsa, which originally came from pagan holidays marking the vernal equinox, now is celebrated as the week of carnival before the Lenten fast begins. *Bliny* play a significant role in the celebrations, both as a symbol of excess before the fast as well as a symbol of perfection in terms of their round shape.

55   The word *blin* is used as an euphemism for "F***", meaning something like "darn" or "crap."

56   Kostroma is an East Slavic fertility goddess, who is usually portrayed as a straw effigy and ceremonially burned during the Shrovetide festival.

57   Tea drinking from saucers.

Great Lenten fast one already abstains from meat) should have been called "*Bliny*" Week by the name of its main ritual dish ("*blin*" is a distorted "*mlin*" or "*mlinets*," that is, a dish made out of ground grain). The "*blin*" is a commemorative dish, but at the same time a life-asserting one. It resembles a burial shroud, but it also feeds you and imparts you with a life force. And when red caviar is folded into the *blin*, it promises life beyond the threshold of death. The *bliny* can be dipped into Slavic sour cream or a mushroom sauce, into sunny honey or melted butter; you can fold them into an envelope-like shape and fill them with various kinds of stuffing, but by themselves they have to be simple and primal with almost zero taste (like water in the desert and bread without additives, like raw oysters and avocado flesh, like brut champagne and clear vodka).

Our *Maslenitsa* is a sister of European Carnival, a similar pagan, pre-Christian festival of the banishment of winter (not the season of the year but the embodiment of the death of nature). Orthodox Christianity transformed *Maslenitsa* into one part of the swing's amplitude – which through the revelry of Maslenitsa festivities and the ensuing Forgiveness Sunday is capable of throwing the congregation straight into Bright Monday, the beginning of Great Lent, and to remind the rest of the people how important it is for every family at least a few times a year to bake *pirozhki* pies and make *bliny* so that our children would not grow up to be freaks of nature.

> *The pan for making the bliny (if you do not have one especially designated for this purpose) must be thoroughly rubbed with large grain salt mixed with butter, heated, and oiled with vegetable oil (you can use a halved onion or a tight wick for this purpose, but to everything else I prefer a cube of salo on a fork; it is non-canonical but effective). The sponge dough (with sugar, salt, milk, water, whipped eggs, and various oils), after it is "brought down" a couple of times, should have a liquid quality like a thin sour cream. The bliny are fried no more than 1 minute on each side, then they are stacked, buttered, and served hot or at least warm (never serve cold*

bliny, there is nothing worse in culinary art than wasted work). Those who are apprehensive about yeast or the word "sponge dough" or anything like that, may simply add the flour to kefir, and even these bliny, simplified but prepared with feeling and understanding come out tender and tasty.

Mushroom sauce for the bliny is prepared as follows: in a deep frying pan or sauté pan fry finely cut champignon mushrooms and lightly sautéed onions for 10 mins. Add chopped garlic, greens, salt and pepper, pour sour cream over the mixture and sauté covered, on low heat, for about 15 min. Put the cooked sauce into a bowl and either spread it over or spoon it onto a blin; roll the blin and eat it. Or you can dip the blin into your own personal bowl. At home no one will criticize you for doing it, but the process is more convenient and tastier with the use of a knife and fork.

Fresh Water Carp

The seas and oceans are salty so their waters keep from becoming stale and so living creatures would not rot in them. It seems even strange that when you find herring it's not immediately pickled in the ocean. Nevertheless, the environment has an effect, and the fish of the sea, crayfish, mollusks, etc. taste as tender as their fresh water brothers in general (if only they are not fat or jelly-like herring, salmonids, or oysters. Unlike them, the fresh water fish, regardless of fleshiness, have an amazingly tender taste which, alas!, is applicable only to freshly caught fish. Freezing it is the kiss of death for it. Because carp is the most popular fresh fish in Russian retail markets, let's discuss it.

Many do not like it because of its unpleasant small fork-like bones along the spine, but the carp is not as black as it is painted and only fishing itself can give you more pleasure than the home-made fish soup made out of carp heads. The tastiest carp are those that weigh 1 to 3 lbs. The carp weighing 4 to 6 lbs. are old fish that stupidly grew in thickness, being transformed into something like a log. On the cutting board stun the live fish and quickly pierce its head with a narrow-tipped knife so it does not flap and suffer. Clear off the scales (but do not throw them away –rinse them with running water), remove the insides and the gills from the fish, rinsing it under a strong stream of water, and divide it into three parts: tails will be used for making the broth, heads – for soup, and the body pieces – for frying, baking in foil, or preparing fish in aspic.

The broth is made out of the tails, scales, root vegetables (onion, carrot, parsley and necessarily celery) and spices (a few bay leaves, a few kernels of allspice, and a dozen black peppercorns, a sprig of parsley, and a sprig of dill), and strain after it is done.

To make the fish soup, add cubed potatoes, 1 Tbsp. of barley and finely chopped fresh or sautéed vegetables, and finally carp heads (the heads are cooked in the lightly boiling broth for not more than 10-15 min, and are ready when the eyes become white and hard). It is advisable to pour a shot of vodka into the cooked fish soup and let it stand covered until it is steeped. When you pour the soup into bowls, sprinkle greens and pepper over it. The real feast is at the bottom of your bowl when in the end you will begin to take apart and chew over the soft-boiled carp's head.

The small fork-like bones are located only along carp's spine and near the tail. Because of this, you will have to remove them by hand together with the spine and ribs after slightly undercooking the fish and spreading it flat into two parts, if you want to make the **fish in aspic***. The fish will reach the right condition after being placed into the dish and covered with the hot salted broth (the same as for the fish soup, but much more concentrated as a result of evaporation) with gelatin and seasoned with small lemon segments, slices of hard-boiled egg, and chopped parsley and celery.*

If you are going to fry the fish, there is an ingeniously simple method for deboning the carp. A chunk of carp is cut lengthwise as deep as these bones and spread out eagle-

like. *In sizzling vegetable oil, the fork-like bones will dissolve without a trace. The juicy carp flesh is accompanied well by white horseradish, white wine, vodka, as well as soy and pomegranate sauces.*

The family of carp includes **Crucian carp** *that are, seemingly on purpose, created for frying on the strength of the absence of the damned small fork-like bones (if such a bone gets stuck in your throat, don't even think of drinking water, try to push it through with chewed up bread). The Crucian carp is a fish fair and square and, as such, it is best to fry it in vegetable oil and then sauté it in sour cream. The frying pan must be sizzling hot, the vegetable oil – heated thoroughly and salted, and the fish – dried out with a paper towel, lightly spiced (with something like Georgian allspice), and rolled in flour. Fry it on high heat and bring it to readiness by simmering it covered in sour cream. The entire process, not counting the preparation, will take 10-15 min. Don't just forget, after you descale and gut the Crucian carp (not bigger in size than the length of your palm) to remove gills sticking out of the heads in order not to spoil the taste of the dish. If the fish is freshly caught or at least not dead, it becomes simply the "music of the spheres" for fishermen, with whom I identify myself.*

Wild Salmon

I had an acquaintance, a Bavarian fish breeder who became rich performing sex change operations – on fish. First he invented a humane method of getting caviar from the salmon and sturgeon without killing the fish – something like a coat with buttons or zipper sewn into the female fish's stomach. You unzip it, unload the caviar, zip it up again, and release the fish back into the stocking pond. Then he went further: he started to transplant sex glands of the red fish into carp, and total surrealism ensued. Just imagine a female carp swimming with Beluga genitalia, which completely lost any idea of what it is. That is why when my photographer friend shared his impressions with me after visiting a Scandinavian farm where they bred "Atlantic salmon for broiling," I somehow completely switched my preferences toward our Northern and Kamchatka salmon, which is much more "wild," skinny, and underdeveloped, but more natural at the same time (at the expense of my taste receptors, I must admit).

*Salmon is good no matter how you cook it; nevertheless, two dishes are absolutely in a class by themselves. The first is **mildly cured salmon**, which the larger and fatter it is, the more oily and tastier it will be, an ideal cold hors d'oeuvre and a good food chaser after drinking vodka. It's very easy to cure the salmon, but there are a few nuances here. Simply sprinkle the filet of salmon with a mixture of stone salt and sugar (not more than 5% of the weight of the fish in a 3:1 proportion) and splash it with cognac or even vodka (that will prevent the formation of the typical "fishy" odor even if you store the dish for a long time) and keep it covered for 2 – 3 days in a cold place (you may put it into the freezer, but the taste will not be as good then).*

*Another wonderful dish is the **solyanka made out of the head of the large Atlantic salmon**, which contains a lot of tender cartilage and jelly-like parts (it goes without saying that before you cook it, you need to remove the gills and also the sharp tabular bones and hard pieces of cartilage). The strained broth is topped off with fish, pickles sautéed in their own brine or sauerkraut, olives, sautéed root vegetables with a small amount of tomato paste, green vegetables and a slice of lemon. But the main nuance is the use of pickled mushrooms, which are capable of transforming the fish solyanka into a real culinary masterpiece. But keep in mind that factory-pickled mushrooms are, more often than not, tasteless. But how to pickle mushrooms for solyanka and cabbage soups on your own, I will explain another time, closer to autumn.*

Kulichi (Easter Cakes) and Dyed Eggs

Even if you don't believe either in God or the devil, try to bake a **kulich** and to dye eggs at least once in your life. This activity will at least make you better because you will do it not for yourself, whom you love over everyone else, but for your family or close friends and will treat them to these dishes. If you follow the recipe, the **kulich** will not come out any worse than one you might buy in a store (in America you can't do it at all, so it is a moot point). Perhaps, it might be even better than in a store because you won't economize for the sake of making it cheaper and will imbue it with your tender feeling for those near and dear to you. Many are a bit afraid of the dough – it is too much trouble: it is capricious, and you need to clean up after making it. But treat it as though it were a living organism, which, in fact it is, thanks to its fresh ingredients and the yeast first of all. Any kind of fermenting fears drafts and requires care and attention. The best conditions for the dough fermenting are a temperature of about 80°F, no direct sunlight or drafts, and peace. There are dozens of recipes for *kulich*, some for showing off *a la* the Russian Betty Crocker Elena Molokhovets, others – without doing that. The optimal one looks approximately like this:

Sift 1 lb. of flour (the process is called "aeration," that is, fluffing the dough with particles of air) – it will be used for making the sponge dough (in other words, the fermented dough that will contain everything except for the fatty and sticky products that hinder the fermenting process). Place the sifted flour into a deep container; add 1 cup of sugar, and ½ tsp of salt. Mix it well, pour in the yeast, diluted in warm milk (2 oz. of the pressed or 1 packet of dry yeast – approximately 1/3 of an oz.), and add another cup of milk. Carefully knead the dough with a wooden spoon and put it in a warm place, covered with a towel. Also put 4 sticks of sweet cream butter in the same warm place for it to soften.

In an hour you may start preparing the sweet base of the kulich. Break 8 eggs, separating the whites from the yolks. Whip both the whites and the yolks (you can use a fork but it will take considerably more time and effort). Mix 1 Tbsp. of each in a separate bowl and save the mixture for later to spread on top of the kulich before putting it into the stove – so that its top would turn reddish like the top of a boletus mushroom. Next add the yolks to the risen sponge dough and knead, then add the butter and knead the mix even more carefully, until the butter is completely dissolved. Add 1Tbsp of vegetable oil, 2 ½ oz. of steamed raisins, 1 packet of vanilla, and a shot glass of cognac or a high quality strong liqueur. Add another 1 lb. of the sifted flour and whipped whites, carefully knead the dough and put it in a warm place under a towel for 1 – 2 hours. During that time, set the risen dough down a couple of times and with the spoon, knead it and allow it to rise again.

The baking container should be cylindrical. Butter it inside with butter or margarine and dust it with cream of wheat, shaking the excess out. It can be a 1 ½ – 2-quart pot, an enamel quart mug, or a ½ quart stainless steel mug – this way you will have an entire Easter family of kuliches. You should fill the containers with dough only up to the half their height or just a little higher so that the head of the risen kulich doesn't push out too much sideways. The kulich is baked in an oven pre-warmed to 400°F for a bit more or less than an hour, depending on the size of the kulich. Try not to open the oven door more than necessary, watching the kulich through the glass door. When the tops of the kulich rise above the top of the containers and acquire a bright yellow or deep brown color, make haste and take the kulich out (you don't even have to check if it's ready with a toothpick). Smooth butter on the top of the kulich, and put it in the baking container on its side. Cover it with the towel and let it cool for 30 min. The kulich should come out easily, but if not, use a fine knife for going along the inner perimeter of the container, turn it upside down, and tap the container on the bottom. To avoid the problem of retrieving the kulich, don't use cream of wheat, but put parchment paper along the wall of the container. Those **kulichi** intended to be consumed with tea may be dusted with powdered sugar; the rest can be eaten with anything you want – from pickled herring to fish in aspic, which represents a special attraction at the Easter table.

Dyed eggs represent the second most important attribute and decoration of the Easter table, which is much more ancient than Easter itself, because it goes all the way back to the mythological image of the "world egg," from which our Universe had hatched and in which all kinds of life have originated. It was a conclusion that our ancestors drew from their observations of surrounding nature. An egg is a symbol of metamorphoses similar to that of the cocoon and butterfly, to yang and yin looking at each other, or life and death pregnant with each other, all of them being involved in an endless cycle and argument – over which comes first and which is more important.

Precisely because of this, eggs are dyed and blessed, that is, imbued with a meaning not usually associated with a simple provision. To paint eggs, to turn them into *pysanky* (as the decorative Easter eggs are called in Ukraine) is entirely an art, which requires special skills, knowledge, practice, the proper instruments, and materials. However, nothing prevents you from making a few simplehearted *"krashenki"* (painted eggs), not the lavishly decorated ones, but just painted all over – for a table decoration. Don't trust paint sets that are sold nowadays before Easter [in Russia], they are usually of a very bad quality and made of God knows what. Garish paper stickers for eggs are nothing but kitsch. Instead use a trusted natural dye – onion skin.

> First hard boil the eggs so they won't crack – do it in a colander dipped in boiling water. Cool them. Cut scotch tape into thin strips. Pick the strip with the tip of a knife and paste them onto the eggs. There are millions of patterns you can use – small crosses along the midsection of the egg, one large St. Andrew's cross,[58] small crosses on both the top and bottom of the

---

[58] Peter the Great introduced the Order of St. Andrew in 1698 as an award for the

egg, etc. Then simmer them for 10 mins with a large amount of onion skin. After you cool the eggs off, take away the Scotch tape and you will find white crosses on brown-colored eggs. If you cook a few of the brown eggs in the same water with the onion skin, they will be dyed into a deep brown color, which is not intrinsic to eggs. These chocolate-colored eggs will only stress and highlight the beauty of the other eggs – the ones with white crosses. When you stack them out of a saucer with a white or embroidered napkin, next to the kulich on a bread board (two more brown hues for you), the eggs will undoubtedly become the main decorative embellishment of your Easter table – stern and simple but, what is of no less importance, made by your own hands.

Pies and *Pirozhki*

After we are no longer fearful of dough, it would be a sin not to indulge your family with pies, especially you women out there. Who does not remember that arousing scent wafting from the kitchen – home forever – mama or grandma is baking pies or fried *pirozhki*! That is the union of mother and oven, next to which the entire family gathers. But the time comes for us to bake pies on our own – no one will do it for us, there must be at least one person in each generation who must know how to bake pies.

The simplest and most traditional Russian pie is of course the enclosed **cabbage pie** or *kulebyaka*. That is, that "stove" from which you start "dancing,"[59] enriching the cabbage filling with mushrooms or hard boiled eggs, or completely replacing it with another – meat, for example (minced boiled meat or chicken with sautéed onions and a little bit of greens, almost without salt), or fish (fried salt-

---

most outstanding military or civilian service. It represents a blue cross in an X-shape with the figure of St. Andrew (the patron saint of the Slavs) crucified on it.

59 Klekh is playing with the saying "plyasat' ot pechki" here, which means "to begin at the beginning" and literally can be translated as "to dance from the stove."

water fish fillet with sautéed onions and parsley, sprinkled with soy sauce), or vegetables (mashed potatoes with fried mushrooms and sautéed onion or even puréed split peas). In this case, the "form" is much more important than the "contents."

The dough is ordinary yeast dough. It is prepared without sponge starter dough because the amount of fat and sweets (eggs and sugar) in it is small. Yeast will be able to "raise" this kind of dough without much difficulty. Sift 1 ½ lbs. of flour, add 1 Tbsp. of sugar, ½ tsp of salt, ¾ cup of milk, ¾ cup of water, 1oz. of pressed yeast diluted in warm milk or ½ of a packet (1/5 oz.) of dried yeast, 2-3 Tbsps. of vegetable oil, and 2 eggs, mix it all well in a deep pot or bowl with a wooden spoon, cover with a towel, and put it in a warm place for 1-2 hours. During that time you will have to press the dough down at least two times and knead it again – this will make the dough more spongy and add some pizzazz to it. After it is ready, the dough is pressed down again and 2/3 of it is placed on a well-buttered baking sheet in the shape of a rectangle, approximately ¾" thick (so that the dough does not sag under the filling). Put the filling on the dough, leaving ¾" free on the edges. For our purposes, let it be cabbage filling consisting of 1 ½ lbs. of cabbage, lightly sautéed with 1 onion, and mixed with 2 chopped hard-boiled eggs, and 1 Tbsp. of diced dill. Add a couple of Tbsps. of hot water and green onions and sauté the mixture covered for about 15 mins. The sides of the pie are pried with a knife or spatula and upturned to form a kind of a trough for filling. You pinch the sides (so they don't sag) with your fingers greased with vegetable oil (so the dough doesn't stick to them). The most important thing is to cover the pie, and you may need an extra pair of hands to do this or extraordinary dexterity. The remaining one-third of the dough must be stretched over the pie like a roof. To do this, flatten the dough in the palms of your hands to the size of a handkerchief, attach one of its edges to the side of the pie and pull it to the other three sides. When you do it, pinch the dough along the entire perimeter. If small rips develop here and there, don't lose heart and try to fix them – the dough is elastic and stretches well. Don't forget too that if you succeed in stretching the top leaf of the dough without rips, you'll have to make several small openings to allow the steam to escape the filling while it bakes.

What's left next is to spread whisked egg (the yoke is the best) over the top of the pie for more intensive browning, let it stand on the stove for 5 – 7 mins, so that the yeast comes back to life, and put it in the oven, warmed up to 360°F. The pie can be taken out in 30 – 40 mins. Check if the pie is ready with a toothpick – it must come out dry after you stick it in the pie (the most important thing is that the bottom should not be mushy, and for that, the filling should not be too moist). The pie is moved by spatulas onto a cutting board, buttered on top (the hot pie absorbs the butter like a sponge), and covered with a paper towel. It is not advisable to eat the pie when it is piping hot. It is fraught with all kind complications for digestion and in some cases can result in intestinal twisting and bowel obstruction. But do not allow the pie to cool down completely either. In 10 – 15 mins you can very well be ready to serve it – cut it into portions and place them on plates. You can spread some butter along the cuts, which will even further enrich its remarkable taste.

Baked pirozhki *(mini pies) are prepared in the same way as the pie, the only difference being that the risen dough is placed on a kneading board and rolled into a "sausage," which is cut into pieces 1 ½ – 2 oz. each (1 ½ lbs. of flour will give you 15 – 20 pirozhki). Place the little cylindrical pieces on end, press them down with the palm of your hand and stretch to get 1/3 of an inch-thick circles. The rest is the same as for baking the pie: the filling is piled on them and the pirozhki pinched to keep them closed; they are placed on a baking sheet with the pinched seam down, smeared with whisked egg (use a soft brush, bird feather, or just your fingers to do that), and placed in the oven. Then they are taken out, buttered, and covered with a towel.*

Just the baking time will be a bit shorter. A good filling for the pirozhki is rice boiled in vegetable or chicken broth diluted in water (the rice-liquid ratio is 1/1 ½ cups) with diced hard-boiled eggs and green onions.

Fried *pirozhki* are a special category. In ancient Rus, the frying process was called "spinning," but our ancestors did not succeed at it. That is why it was not a sin to borrow some practices from Turkish kitchens together with some dishes – such as *cheburek* (a kind of meat calzone) and *belyash* (a meat pastry).

Belyashi, *to keep them from being coarse, require an ultrathin dough, which should literally run through your fingers and threaten to spill onto the floor. To handle it, spread a little oil onto your hands, put a piece of dough on floured kneading dough, and quickly form a 6" diameter circle; drop a heaped Tbsp. of filling onto it, and pinch the dough, leaving it 1 ½" – 2" in diameter on top. The dough is the same as for the cabbage pie but twice as thin (reduce the amount of flour and eggs by 20-30% and increase for the same the amount of liquid and yeast).*

The filling is salted, and peppered ground beef with a large amount of onions, parsley, and a few cloves of garlic are mixed together (unlike the filling for the cabbage pie, the filling for belyashi should be relatively moist and juicy). Belyashi are fried quickly on high heat in a deep frying pan in a large amount of lightly salted vegetable oil – be sure to keep your eyes open: fry for one minute with the opening down, and one minute with the opening up, and the cooked belyash then is transferred into a deep covered bowl. As soon as the burned flour has accumulated on the bottom of the pan, drain the oil to a different pan and continue to fry the belyashi in it (or you can drain the oil into a different container, quickly wipe the burnt flour off the bottom of the pan, return the oil back to the pan, and continue frying). In both cases let the oil warm up once again. Belyashi go well with a sauce. The classic one is made with wine vinegar, which is poured into the opening of the belyash. **Tomato sauce for ground beef**, *prepared quickly, is also quite good with them: 3 ½* *oz. of tomato paste, ½ tsp of Georgian adjika sauce, 1 large clove of crushed garlic, thinly chopped dill, parsley, and definitely cilantro; and finally boiled water or beef broth for diluting the sauce to the right consistency.*

From the thicker dough (it will be thinner than for the cabbage pie, but not as thin as for the *belyashi*), you can make **fried *pirozhki*** filled with mashed potatoes and onions sautéed on *salo*, which are more customary and natural for Russian people. The cooking method is the same as for *belyashi*, but please remember that water dripping into the scorching oil can result in serious burns for you.

Cabbage – it is the Head!

There are dozens of kinds of cabbage in the world, and each is good in their own way. The curly Savoy cabbage is good in European soups; the pale Peking cabbage – in Chinese salads with wood mushrooms; Brussels sprouts, sautéed in batter, as a side dish; red cabbage – marinated; and young green kohlrabi (cabbage-turnips), which in taste resembles a stalk of white cabbage or the stems of cauliflower, in soups or raw, with a mayonnaise dressing.

Nevertheless, the head (pun intended) of all cabbages is the traditional green one, the juiciest and most universal, which is good in salads, in soups, in main courses, and for marinating. It is especially good twice a year – early and late (when after the first frost the juices go to its head, and that is the best time for it to be pickled).

I never liked the tired emigrant witticism about early strawberries that come up for sale at 6 in the morning and not at the end of May, because, I repeat, nothing makes food more appealing than when it's in season. In the same way, nothing can compare to the finesse of the taste of the first curly head of young green cabbage, the messenger of approaching summer.

The simplest vegetable soup with it and a tablespoon of butter, without any meat, is already something, and if you add miniature meatballs to the soup – it's super good! However, without a doubt you should also cook this early cabbage before it becomes mature once in a while to prepare *golubtsy* (stuffed cabbage leaves), or properly speaking – *"golubchiks,"* the very name of which brings associations with turtledoves.[60]

> *In the beginning you will have to struggle with the cabbage leaves that have grown into each other and then keep them covered in boiling water for five minutes. For the filling: mix equal parts of ground beef, sautéed with onions and carrots, and semi-ready rice, cooked in water, and chicken or vegetable broth (1/1 ¼ proportion), add parsley, cilantro, salt and pepper to taste. Dissolve sour cream and 1 Tbsp. of tomato paste in the cabbage broth. Place the filling onto the cabbage leaves and roll them. Put the golubtsy in the broth, drop a couple of bay leaves into it, cover them with a plate, cover the pot, and cook at medium heat for 40 mins. If you make golubtsy using mature cabbage, sauté it before putting the cabbage leaves in the pot. The taste of the golubtsy is made even better with all kinds of "additives" – such as sweet peppers or a few prunes. The golubtsy have to sit half-drowning in the sauce when they are put on a plate with sour cream and greens (dill, parsley, cilantro) spooned on top of it. Golubtsy are a strictly family dish – so arm yourself with a spoon and bread and shamelessly attack the sauce until it's all gone.*

You can read about everyday cabbage soup, *bigos*, cabbage pie, and sauerkraut in other parts of this book.

Smooth Jams and Lazy Preserves

Many nations cook fruit and berries with sugar and preserve them. Anglo-Saxons prefer jam, the continental Europeans – *comfiture* (refined jam with the addition of jellying pectin, which allows for the reduction of sugar content as a conserving agent), the Ukrainians –

---

60 In original Russian the word *golubchik* literally means "little dove" (masc.), *golubka* is the feminine noun for she-dove or turtle-dove.

their fruit butter, Russians – their preserves. Where you have an excess of sunlight, you will find an excess of sugar in fruit – that is why in the south fruits are simply sun- and air-dried either as whole or pressed, ending up with "dry jam." Each of the products has its plusses and minuses. Our preserves are over-sweetened and require tea the way a carriage needs a horse. But no comfiture or dried apricot has such a tender taste and head-spinning scent as properly cooked Russian preserves. And the more tender the "raw material," the more killer of a scent you get. Our mothers already didn't know how to make preserves the way our grandmothers did (they knew some secret that consisted of, perhaps, the freshness of the berries, or, perhaps, in the fact that the strawberries were dipped in cognac or vodka before being cooked, although I don't remember that now. You didn't have to bring their preserves to your nose to smell them; it was enough just to take the cover off.

Generally speaking, however, one of the well-known secrets is like it is in the old Russian saying: "plenty is no plague" – an excess of sugar intensifies and better preserves the berries' aroma (the proportion must be 1½:1 and not 1:1). **Strawberries** *or* **raspberries** *are covered with half the amount of sugar and placed in the refrigerator for a night where they should release their juice. We use this juice and the remaining sugar to cook the syrup, into which we carefully thrust the berries (without stirring, just carefully shaking the pot!). We bring the preserves to a boil, skim the top, and let it cool for a few hours. And we have to repeat the process several times – only then are the tender berries cooked without overcooking. They are not supposed to lose their color and form, but become semi-transparent and be immersed in the transparent syrup. If the berries float to the surface or sink to the bottom, it would be a catastrophe. You may add a pinch of lemon juice and lemon peel into the syrup to strengthen the smell and color, and to prevent mold and saccharification. The preserves are poured slightly warm into sterilized jars with screw-on lids.*

A Georgian woman from whom I used to buy huge dark red Cornelian cherries told me the secret of amazing **Cornelian cherry preserves**, which our Russian cooks seem to know only how to spoil.

> *It turns out that it in order for the berries not to become wrinkled and hard, they should be cooked no longer than 15 minutes, then they turn out sweet and sour and jelly-like (2 lbs. of berries cooked in syrup made of 2 lbs. of sugar and 1 cup of water)!*

And here is a way to prepare a stunning **plum** (or **apricot**) marmalade, which I personally perfected and in which I take great pride. I remember how the Carpathian Hutsuls, smoking their pipes, tirelessly stirred cooking plums in huge vats all day long.

> *They told me the proportion – 1/10 of the amount of sugar of the weight of pitted plums (preferably purple ones with a whitish coating) without a drop of water. But there is no way I will stick around cooking plums all day long! And it dawned on me: in order for the marmalade not to burn, it must be cooked bathed in water for two days (that way the marmalade thickens better). In principle it can be cooked to a consistency that it can be cut with a knife. What pressed jam can compare with this kind of marmalade!*

Is eggplant really "blue"?

Adjika, Adjab-Sandal (eggplant and vegetable ragout), Eggplant, *Imam-Bayildi* (baked stuffed eggplant), or the Culinary ABCs of the East

The East about which I will be writing is located to the south of Russia. It is a geographic area where there is enough sunlight for the good growth of "Blue Ones" as our ladies of the house call the eggplant. However, this is not everything; there is also a subtle "Muslim" taste that dominates the products cultivated in that South and dishes made from them. For example, eggplant and various southern herbs grow in the south of Russia and in Ukraine, but as a result of some secret collusion, they migrate to influence Turkic and Circassian cuisines. Eggplant and sweet pepper for us are still "twice removed" relatives, although we should have stopped shunning away from them and unnecessarily waste the products. A Russian person as well as a Ukrainian will eat eggplant, but without really putting his or her soul into it, tormenting it, not allowing the eggplant to fully reveal its taste – he will put it in a press and squeeze out its sourness, then, after rolling it in flour, fry it cut into circles, and gobble it up; or "grind" it into what we call "eggplant caviar." It should not be that way, and not everyone does it this way.

In some way Russia is a subcontinent, almost equal to Asia in its vastness, and being capable of absorbing and assimilating products and dishes with the most unusual, it would seem, taste (not to look far for an example, think about "tops and roots"[61] – potatoes and tomatoes; or sunflowers, which used to be considered a kind of weed until people fell in love with husking sunflower seeds, and some *kurkul* (a rich Ukrainian peasant), after many years of futilely trying to find some use for it, stumbled into the idea of extracting sunflower oil from it. Open-mindedness toward the foreign is intrinsic for developed culinary cultures and all the more constitutes a characteristic feature of those we can call a kind of culinary empire – the Great French, or the "Mediterranean" one; the Chinese; and immediately following it Russian-Great-Russian (please forgive my unsubstantiated rating of the great cuisines because each of them is ingenious in its own right, I am speaking only about the inertia or flexibility of principles, about a sharp delineation of transparency). But enough stipulations, let's move to the matter at hand.

There are different kinds of *adjikas*. The *Soviet adjika*, consisting of 90% salt, wasn't bad in some respects, but was good only as an

---

61 A reference to a Russian folktale, in which a peasant and a bear share crops by one of them taking the "tops" and the other – the "roots" (with the peasant every time tricking the bear into taking an unfavorable share: the first year they share a crop of beets, with the bear taking the tops and the peasants the "roots," the second year it is wheat in the reverse order...).

addition to the end product. The universally loved Caucasian *adjika* differs from that one by less salt content, but it is primarily oriented to the dishes of the Caucasus cuisines and as a result of this, doesn't find widespread use at the Great-Russian table. There is one more *adjika*, which Russian homemakers love to produce in large volume. The fact that it can be eaten with a tablespoon is both to its merit and a shortcoming. As a condiment for borsht, it is quite good, but as an independent sharply piquant sauce for the majority of meat dishes, it is not. The main problem is the tomatoes, with which women start to prepare this kind of *adjika*. They have a beautiful bright red color, but what about the acid, the seeds, and this penchant for fermenting? No, think what you will, but I am forever an aficionado of the **Crimean-Tartar *adjika*** in which, instead of the dubious tomatoes, red sweet pepper (which is also a champion among the vitamin-bearing veggies) is used.

Here is the recipe: Use 2 lbs. of meaty red pepper and 3-4 chili peppers. Clean both peppers of seeds (don't forget that the stinging of the pepper will be transferred to your fingers, no matter how vigorously you rub them off and wash; therefore, don't even think about touching your eyes or a tender spot on your skin with them for about two hours – when you figure out what is happening to you, it already will be too late). Prepare 12 oz. of garlic and greens – a sprig of dill, a sprig of parsley, half of that of coriander, and/or celery, and a small sprig of basil (the smell and taste of the last two are very vivid, therefore, their introduction into the bouquet requires tact and a sense of measure).

Grind everything listed above – it is up to you how you are going to do it, but remember that the standard meat grinder will kill a considerable amount of the vitamin C, which is not desirable). Moderately salt (1-2 tsps) the resulting green-red mixture and place it into tightly closed glass jars. Find a place for them in your refrigerator – at a low temperature, the adjika will not ferment and nothing will happen to it. Keep one jar of adjika for everyday use.

Every time you open it, you'll understand that you did right by refusing to pasteurize and can the "base product," and in doing so, preserving all the vitamins as well as a spicy fresh aroma that momentarily spreads all over the room, that is capable of causing profuse salivation even from a corpse as well as the desire to immediately come to life and demand a tenderized pork chop, and to send the recently spawned preachers of "right eating" running every which way. Those who try to prepare the *adjika* in the above-mentioned way will forever refuse to add tomatoes to it.

The taste of **tkemali** *(Georgian plum sauce for meat dishes), which is equally good for meat, fish, and vegetable dishes, is also simply remarkable. Tkemali plums or sour cherry plums are the best to prepare it. Cook it in an enameled vat bathed in water the same way as you would plum marmalade (see the Index). When the skin, flesh, and pits are divided in the cherry-plum mass, cool it off and squeeze the resulting mash through a sieve. Add crushed garlic, sugar, salt, and pepper to taste, and also a small quantity of greens (but considerably less than for the adjika).*

Another short recipe: **lobio** *(a Georgian kidney bean dish), a dish that the Russians love so much, but for some reason do not cook themselves. Cook red (brown, pinto, or any kind, except white) beans. Drain the broth, but do not discard it - it can be eaten as a soup or used in preparing sauces. Finely chop onions (you can use green onions, too), pepper, salt, and sprinkle it with vinegar, add vegetable oil, and mix everything. The dish is ready. It can be eaten as a salad or as a side dish for meat, with pasta and rice (then it will be Armenian pilaf lobi-chilav, because any loose rice by itself is considered to be a "pilaf" in many nationalities – the base model and the zero-degree of it).*

Now it is time to start talking about **eggplant**, which only looks "blue" from the outside, not to mention the fact that ripe eggplant must be blue-black in color, and its fleshy sides should shine like the sides of a chestnut horse. The eggplant is good in all forms and methods of cooking, but it reaches its peak and the innermost capabilities of its taste – and I insist on this – by being baked. "Reinventing the wheel, aren't you" – the male and female lovers of the "blue ones" will say. I'll answer: not reinventing, but just confirming and testifying to it. At the same time I think it is a fatal mistake to bake the eggplant in an oven, in which they first puff up like blimps and then burst like light bulbs, while remaining undercooked. The eggplant must be baked only on charcoal. It is also incredibly beautiful: when before bringing out the skewed *basturma* (pastrami)-*khorovats* (vegetable shish kebab)-shish kebab for a sacrifice, similar swords with crimson hearts of tomatoes, green peppers skewered side-ways, and the heavy, sweating silky bodies of eggplants with their sagging backs lie on the calescent coals.

In a home kitchen we'll have to achieve this result on the equivalent of coals – on a sizzling-hot round metal sheet or a large cast-iron frying pan, carefully rubbed clean and wiped dry. The eggplant must be charred black on all sides. Turning it as its skin gets charred bit by bit, you'll end up with an eggplant that will look like a cut-glass decanter and that you'll have to place on one end and bake same this way, too. Transferring it onto a cutting board or a plate, you'll now be able, having pried it with a knife, to unbutton it and take off the stiff, charred skin all at once, like a coat. The tender steaming flesh of the bare eggplant will make your nostrils involuntarily enflame. Make a single stroke with a knife and chop off a slice of the lower seeded part and, burning your fingertips, dip its edge into salt. Put it on your tongue. You don't have to close your eyes – you'll never forget this moment. You'll never in your life confuse the taste of **baked eggplant** *with something it's not.*

This, however, is not the pinnacle of flavor, and we will try to surpass it.

Bake a half dozen of eggplants, the same number of green peppers, and one ripe tomato until its skin is clearly burned and blackened. Skin them all and remove the seeds from the *peppers. Incidentally, it must be said, that I recently began to keep the seeds because they add a piquant taste and are good for the digestive system (by the way, if you dry out and grind these seeds, you'll get a white powder with the remarkably consistent scent of green pepper for your winter sauces). After that, dice the flesh of the baked vegetables with bold strikes of the knife. Meanwhile, sauté onions in vegetable oil until they are golden brown, then mix them with the baked vegetables, and sauté covered for about 10 mins. Add a few cloves of crushed garlic, finely chopped dill, parsley, and cilantro to the mixture. Salt it lightly and mix it well. You may also sprinkle it with vinegar and add a bit of a non-refined vegetable oil (especially if you want to keep it in a jar for a few days as a cold appetizer). Cover the frying pan and simmer it for five more minutes. When the pan cools down, transfer the mixture into a jar and cool it more in the refrigerator. That will be the best of all imaginable **eggplant caviars**, which only you can cook. Now cut a slice of white bread, spread butter on it, and pile it up with the caviar. Of all vegetable appetizers this will be the best one. And if you want, you can use the eggplant caviar as a side dish – for example, for shish kebab (without any burned rings of onion and tomato circles! You have to remember that the onions, which have served for the marinade and given all their juice to the meat, are always discarded). In the Caucasus, this kind of warm caviar is picked up by a piece of lavash (Georgian pita) bread as a side or sauce for the shishkebab. Men grill meat and bake vegetables, women prepare the caviar. No hard feelings all around. And only a caviar like this deserves the heralded title of "our own caviar."*

However, we are more accustomed to the taste of the fried eggplant in a purely vegetable or meat ragout. It is the eggplant that imparts the characteristic coloring and determines the taste range of such famous Caucasian dishes as **adjab-sandal** or **imambayaldy** (literally, the "imam-got-high" – tried it and fainted, as the legend says. Whoever said it, he was a holy person, although such a notion of saintliness is somewhat difficult for us to evaluate.). It is principally a Turkic or, perhaps, Turkish dish, and the Bulgarian-Moldovan moussaka is a Balkan version of the same "imam-got-high."

Add the eggplant, the sweet and spicy peppers, zucchini, tomatoes, garlic, and piquant greens into our ragout of the sautéed ribs with root greens, potatoes, and sour cream, and you will understand what he got high on. It is better to stew this ragout in an oven in a covered clay pot for at least an hour, or in a covered goose dish at worst. You can always find a solution.

The Kitchen of a Hot Summer Day

Summer forces us to use the stove more rarely and the refrigerator – more often. Woe to a person caught in a city apartment by the arrival of the summer heat, especially if the city is a megalopolis and your house is built out of cement blocks, which means that it takes two or three days after the weather changes for it to cool off. During a sleepless night, under the militant buzzing of mosquitoes, when the temperature in the apartment does not go below 90°F, and there is no foreseeable end to it, I always recall a concise statement by my old friend in infinite correctness, of which I never cease to be convinced.

It just happened that, by force of various circumstances, he and I lived for almost a year at a Moscow countryside *dacha* that belonged to one of our common acquaintances. The winter that year turned out to be severe – in December a -30°F cold hit. The working AGV heating system just warmed the water in the pipes not allowing them to freeze. The uninsulated walls of the *dacha* shuddered and yielded to the will of the frost that gripped the area. Even the mice grew quiet in them and the cockroaches disappeared. For a few days my friend and I stayed in our beds, having pulled on all the winter clothes we had and thrown on all the blankets we were able to find on the first floor. We didn't have any inkling of going to the city, going to work, or doing something useful.

The only thing that worried me a little was that my friend did not get up for a few days even for going to the outhouse, not to mention to get something to eat or cook something. Despite my childhood memory of the Yenisei[62] cold, I understood a lot of things in Russian history – I felt it with my own skin, to the bones – I understood what happened to Napoleon and his army, and what happened to Hitler and his division in Moscow and on the Volga. In any case, when I, unable to conquer my human nature, intended once again to hop outside, my friend suddenly called to me from under the heap of blankets. Fighting his teeth from chattering, but with the enormous power of conviction, he forced out, and I barely understood it: "Anyway, it's be-be-tter than, tha-n 90°F in the shade."

He grew up in Saratov and knew what he was talking about – while preparing for the entrance exam to Saratov University he had to lie up to his neck in a bathtub filled with cold water. After all, the frigid cold is outside, if worse comes to worst, you can burn the *dacha* to get warm. For a warm-blooded creature the heat is much more intolerable, because to cool yourself on the inside when the heat is nested in an overheated body, appears to be an impossible task. However, the most unpleasant thing in the sultry weather is to catch cold from all kinds of artificial drafts and excessively over-chilled drinks. The more so that, as peoples who are much more savvy in enduring the heat know, not every drink helps you endure it. The heat (just like alcohol) washes out all kinds of nutrients and minerals out of your organism, and the drinks that do not recharge the organism with minerals, being thus a self-deception, make the situation only worse.

Every Russian knows about Kalmyk tea with milk and fat, which looks like fruit pulp and quenches the thirst perfectly, but not everyone will drink it. Green tea is also great in this respect, and also because you can brew it multiple times, but you shouldn't overdo it, or at least don't drink liters of it. Nowadays Americans

---

62 The Yenisei River area in Siberia.

use all kinds of bottled ice tea with different flavors and fragrances – undoubtedly it's better than Coke or Pepsi, but still it's rather a tribute to fashion and customs (especially if we remember that in most American eateries at any time of the year you'll be served a pitcher or at least a glass of filled with ice, and only then do they take your order, as though everyone had grown up in the desert). But it would be cruel, after doing a number on the reader's head, to let him to die from thirst on a hot day.

The remedy that helps quench thirst during the heat of the day and restores energy has been invented long time ago. It's called *ayran*. The simplest *ayran* is *katyk* (a Turkish sour milk drink) or fermented milk, diluted with cold water or water with ice. Recently you can find many drinks sold under by this name, but it's not difficult to prepare its equivalent on your own using products at hand. It's difficult to believe that thirst can be quenched with the help of… garlic and dill (although there is nothing surprising about it – the motto of the drink is "to nurture and not to give a drink"). The Soviet builders of the Aswan Dam in Egypt taught my old friend a long time ago, and he passed it along to me.

> *You can easily make reduced fat sour milk by fermenting milk that is sold in plastic packets with the crust of dark rye bread. The milk sold in the Tetra Pak cartons, which has become so popular with our people, first of all, is not really milk, and secondly, it's not good for fermenting because of the great number of preservatives. Add crushed garlic and finely chopped fresh dill into the sour milk (some also like to add a few crushed caraway seeds or ground mint leaf, and a pinch of salt). Mix all the ingredients well and foam the sour milk with a strong stream of sparkling water, preferably ice cold. Siphons have long gone out of use, but everyone knows the kind of pressure you can achieve by shaking an ordinary bottle of sparkling mineral water vigorously and opening it with your thumb on the top. What is left is to direct the stream at the sour milk, gradually releasing your thumb. The accidental splashing will also have a refreshing effect. One pint of the ayran, prepared this way,*

brings the most heat-exhausted person back to a normal condition. The mixture can be prepared beforehand in a large quantity and kept in the refrigerator. Separately you can keep, as its "igniter," a battery of sparkling water in glass bottles, preferably domestic ones.

It is appropriate here to say a few words about our native **okroshka** (a cold *kvas* soup with chopped vegetables and meats).

Kvas. *The bottled kvas is more often than not too sweet and abundant with damned additives that are supposed to "improve the taste," and also with stabilizers and preservatives. It is preferable to use the kvas on tap, which is sold from cisterns in the streets, or if worse comes to worst, to make it by yourself using dried black rye bread, sugar and yeast, but this method will require a lot of patience and dedication like that of moonshiners. It is easier to prepare robust kvas out of a concentrate, which is sold everywhere (and the thicker it is the better). For a more active fermenting you can toss a handful of raisins into the mash. You can also prepare the okroshka using the bottled ayran or the whey strained from the sour milk and cooled down.*

There are lovers of such an *okroshka* "diet," but it does not possess the merriment that is imparted to the soup by the swarming *kvas* bubbles that burst in the sour cream when you stir it with a spoon and when the entire surface of the soup moves as if it were alive, from one side of the bowl to another.

Potatoes. *Keep in mind that the skin of true young potatoes must flake and be smeared with earth and not covered with some imitation of it, nothing has changed here. Avoid imported potatoes, washed by shampoos and genetically modified on top of everything, that just pretend to be "young potatoes" (as the strawberries compared to potatoes by their density and other things). Old potatoes should be cooked "in their jackets" (unpeeled) like for a salad. Then add a hardboiled egg, cucumber, green onions, and greens; instead of salt use pickle brine, and finally, an important detail, radishes. Such* *a culinary authority as Pokhlebkin unequivocally despised all who put radishes in the okroshka. He said that the density of the radishes contrasts with that of other components, and an analogous result can be achieved by adding a small amount of horseradish and mustard into the okroshka. Who can argue against the necessity of these two ingredients in the okroshka, but what will we do about the color? We should remember how the white circles and semi-circles with a red rim adorn the okroshka. And the radish's sharp taste is precisely what is needed, and the density will "sag" if you cut the radish into really thin slices – then so much of the crunching that gladdens the soul will remain.*

And now comes the music of the spheres, the stepbrother of the okroshka and vinaigrette, so-called **meatless soup** *or* **cold beet soup***. It includes: cooked "in their jackets" potatoes and finely chopped beets, a pickle, a hardboiled egg, green onions, greens, shredded horseradish, lemon juice, pickle brine, and bread kvas.*

Try it and you'll forget about *okroshka*.

Salads: Advices and Recipes

Do as you like, but there is something dubious about salads, something non-traditional and "heretical" for Russian cuisine. The very word "salad" is borrowed from the Italians and French, and means salted and spiced raw greens. For us, vinaigrette made of cooked vegetables with a spicy dressing is closer; "vinaigrette" is also a Romance word (from *"vinaigre,"* that is, vinegar), although the French call their vinaigrettes "Russian salads." The matter is not in the malicious fine meshing and mixing of the products, which are well known to the Russian culinary practitioners at least through making the *okroshkas* (from the words *"krokha"* [crumb] and *"kroshit'"* [to mince]), but in the use of raw products and vinegar. However, tastes change, and it is long forgotten how our ancestors rioted against potatoes and did not know what to do with sunflowers and tomatoes. But who will dare today to claim that the **salad Olivier**, invented by a 19th century French restaurateur named Olivier in Moscow, is not one of the beautiful principle dishes of Russian cuisine?

It is sort of a meat vinaigrette (because cooked and canned products are dressed with a vinegar-mustard-oil-egg suspension). It's true that the salad suffered greatly in the years of the Soviet public cafeteria system, but there is nothing easier than to return it to its initial appearance. All you have to do is to replace the baloney type of sausage with cooked meat (veal or chicken), the green peas – with capers, and the brine dripping pickles – with the more solid marinated ones. Those who have not tried it will be astounded at how much this simple change can transform and ennoble the universally loved salad Olivier.

Another vinaigrette masterpiece of the Russian table is also of foreign origin – **herring under a coat**, a dish that clearly came to be under the influence of the Jewish kitchen (as pickled herring itself was a Dutch invention that found its most ardent admirers among the Russian people). A paradox consists of the fact that it is not at all easier to find the right fatty pickled herring under capitalism as it was under Socialism, because only the waste of the catch ends up in Russia, and even those are no longer salted in the open sea or at least at seaside factories. By the addresses of the producers you will see that unthawed herring is salted mostly in the dry-land areas of Russia, and this has a devastating effect on its consistency and taste. Various tiny pieces of herring fillet under all kinds of sauces can be of a tender consistency, but as a rule have an insipid taste and are in fact an imitation of the real taste of herring (almost like "crab sticks"[63]). On the other hand, even in Norway recently I was not able to find a decent herring – the same scraggly trash as we have in Russia, and on top of that, it is over-salted or, in the German manner, is sold ready for use with all kinds of fragrances, sauces, and foreign tastes. So the search for a fatty herring turns into a real

---

63 Crab sticks are imitation crab meat sold packed in small cellophane-wrapped rolls.

hunt. But the herring under a coat is good because to prepare it you won't need herring of the highest quality.

Back to business. For two mid-size herring, boil 2 potatoes in their skins, 1 beet, and 1 large carrot. The herring is cleaned and minced with a knife and placed on a plate. Finely chop a medium-size onion and place the first layer of the "coat" over the herring. In a similar way, the cooked vegetables are cut and placed in layers over the herring. If you prefer, instead of cutting the vegetables, you may grate them. Each layer is covered with mayonnaise, or you can put just one thicker layer on top. It would be good to keep the prepared dish in the refrigerator for half an hour – during that time the layers will absorb each other's taste. Obviously it is easier to serve this salad with a spatula like a cake.

As for **fresh summer salads** with vegetable oil (for example, tomatoes and cucumbers with onions, garlic and greens), replace ordinary vinegar with dark balsamic vinegar, and you will feel the direct heat of "food lightning" in your stomach (as the unforgettable W. W. Pokhlebkin put it). If you are looking for a vinegar that you can drink like wine, the Italians in Modena produce it (Aceto Balsamico de *Modena*); today you can buy it in any supermarket.

And here is a recipe for fresh **Chinese salad** *year round. Its main ingredient is the black or white Chinese* **wood mushrooms** *(don't confuse them with shitake mushrooms) that look like cartilaginous ears. They are sold dried or pressed into briquettes (in the latter case you will need to pour boiling water over them and simmer covered until they completely absorb the water; also, remove what would seem like hard roots for you), or you can buy them from Chinese sellers at markets ready-made. By themselves these mushrooms are almost tasteless; their main benefit is consistency and crunch. A royal taste is imparted to them by their "retinue," which includes finely cut* **Peking salad, leeks,** *and young* **zucchini** *(if you don't have it, use cabbage, green onions, and cucumbers);* **sesame seed oil** *(or any other vegetable oil),* **lemon juice** *(from one squeezed lemon), soy* *sauce (or salt), sugar, and ground white (or in the worst case, black) pepper, 1 tsp of sodium glutamate (it looks like sugar or large grain salt and is sold in packets at the Asian food stores and is just as essential as the wood mushrooms). The refreshing taste of this all-weather and moderately exotic salad will, no doubt, astound not only you but also your guests.*

*The number of **all-season salads** also include such primitive dishes as green onions with hardboiled eggs mixed with mayonnaise (adding cucumber and the greens will not hurt it either) or shredded turnip celery with shredded apple mixed in an improvised proportion with mayonnaise. These are sorts of tests of the presence of winter vitamin deficiency – if you suddenly find these salads terribly tasty, make the consequent conclusions. Very close to them stand fruit salads that you can make year round: with oranges, bananas, fresh or frozen strawberries, apples, and kiwi fruit hash served with ice cream or sour cream; or shredded cooked (or even better, baked) beets mixed with soaked and finely cut prunes and crushed walnuts, dressed with sour cream.*

Five More Kinds of Soup

Green *Shchi* (cabbage soup) or **Sorrel Soup**. It is an essential source of vitamin C, which completely satisfies the "sour inclination" of Russian cuisine. It's prepared with a base of meat bouillon or water, with the addition at the very end of a tablespoon of butter. It's also good with tiny croquettes (ground beef mixed with onions and greens, with salt and pepper, cook for 15-20 minutes). Toss diced potatoes and a bay leaf into the salty water or bouillon. In a frying pan sauté chopped yellow onions, carrots, parsley root, stalks of greens and sorrel, and toss into the soup when ready. No earlier than five minutes before turning off the stove, toss in chopped sorrel stalks. The prepared soup is covered and should sit for about five minutes. The soup should be garnished in bowls with chopped round pieces of egg, sour cream, and greens. It couldn't be quicker or simpler, and the main thing – you can eat this kind of soup all year round.

To save time and labor, in the summer you can make the sorrel seasoning for the soup and store it in canning jars (because of the acidity of sorrel in salted form, it will not turn sour or spoil). Sort the sorrel, wash it, then chop it up with a knife. First toss the chopped up stalks into a small amount of boiling water. They will turn brown before your eyes. After a few minutes toss in the sorrel leaves. They also will turn brown and become many times smaller in volume. Cook everything for just a few minutes covered, after which with a slotted spoon transfer the pulp into a clean dry jar, layered with rock salt (use as much of it as you would use for a pot of soup), then pour in the broth and a tablespoon of hot vegetable oil. Screw on the top and store the prepared sorrel filling in a cabinet at room temperature. Any time of year in a half hour you can prepare a fantastic vitamin soup with it. Just don't forget that it's already salted!

During mushroom season take advantage of the circumstances and don't skimp on **Boletus mushrooms** *for the soup: cook them with an onion and bay leaf, let it boil for 20 minutes on low, also toss a single large potato and a handful of grain (barley, buckwheat, or rice) into the hot bouillon, season it with sautéed greens and lighten it in the bowl with sour cream and sprinkle greens over it – you can faint from its scent alone, you'll swallow your tongue from the rich taste of the broth and eat till your heart's content! After all, the Boletus mushrooms have more caloric content than any meat, and no other mushrooms grow next to them.*

Now three winter soups. **Rassolnik** *(sour pickle soup) requires boiled beef kidney. Separate all the fat from the kidney, rinse it well, and cook it on high heat in a large saucepan for 15 minutes (so that the kidney doesn't stick to the bottom and burn, place a straining spoon or a spatula under it). You can add a spoonful of vinegar. The kidney will decrease about to 1/3*

> *of its original size, harden, and release a bunch of bad-tasting thickened foam – you can flush the foam down the toilet, and wash off the liver with cold water. Boil water, put a diced potato into it, a little bit of barley or rice, and the kidney cut up in small, narrow strips, and also a bay leaf, a pinch of black pepper and a few pungent peppercorns. In another pot sauté chopped up tiny bits of pickles salted in their own brine (that's why you won't have to salt the rassolnik), and in a frying pan make a sauté of the roots and stalks of greens (just don't overcook them – when the onions turns brownish red, and the greens soften, splash them with hot water and braise them in a covered pot on low heat). Place the sauté into the soup when it's ready, and when the potato is ready, pour in the pickle seasoning (otherwise the potato will harden in the acidic environment and won't quite be cooked). Let the rassolnik sit with the lid on, covered with a towel. Put sour cream, finely chopped fresh greens, and a black pepper mill on the table. There are other types of rassolnik, but this is the tastiest one.*

A properly cooked **split pea soup** can also be divinely delectable. For this you'll need a shank of meat, raw or smoked. But the first thing you need to do is soak split peas overnight – because the success of this soup depends on whether you are able to cook it close to the consistency of a puree, but not quite a puree – so that it be al dente.

> *So: in the morning pour a large quantity of cold water over the soaked peas with a shank of meat and cook it uncovered on low heat. Toss into that skinned onions, carrots, and parsley root (the cooked greens will be removed from the prepared bouillon after a few hours, and instead of them a new sauté is introduced from those same roots along with stalks of greens). When the peas are half cooked and the meat is just about ready, the soup is salted. Add chopped up potatoes, smoked kielbasa sausage, chopped up in small cubes, several bay leaves, and about ten crushed peppercorns. For this kind of soup it is advisable to prepare crispy croutons made of white French*

bread, cut up in cubes and slightly browned on a grill or in an oven. The croutons are tossed in small portions onto the plate to keep them crunchy. Sour cream isn't necessary, but chopped dill for the soup and mustard for the softness of the shank would be a perfect addition.

But at times it becomes somewhat cramped in the predictable circle of Slavic soups and sometimes you feel like eating wild fare. **Bozbash**, the most refined variety of steppe *ciorba* (a Turkish high fat-content soup made with the previously sautéed meat and vegetables) or a tangy restaurant *kharcho*, as it is impossible to better respond to the desire to diversify the soup repertoire. The main peculiarity of this line of fatty and sour-spicy soups is the fact that it includes mutton, which is not only boiled, but also fried, and also contains fruits and robust acidifiers (from pomegranate or lemon juice, to wine vinegar).

The Russian version of bozbash is made something like this: boil mutton brisket with ribs for about an hour and a half with vegetable roots on low in an uncovered pot; take it out and fry it in a frying pan to a crust and return it into the broth; throw diced potatoes into a pot, a handful of rice and several prune pits; add a large yellow onion, cut up and fried with flour, and then sautéed with tomatoes or tomato paste and spices (pepper – red, greens – coriander) in a deep covered frying pan; acidify the bozbash with the juice of half a lemon. As someone joked back in the last century: thoroughly scratch any Russian – and you'll find a Tartar underneath. But I must confess, that in Asia they know a thing or two about of food. You can read about pilaf in another chapter.

Polenta, or in another word – It's *Mamalyga*

Corn became a part of our table only in cooked form, with salt and a little butter, or husked in cans, used in salads with any kind of "crab sticks" made out of bluefish. Too bad. There is an amazing dish from Roman kitchens, which in Italy is called **polenta**, and in Moldova *mamalyga*. Its single deficiency is that it requires ripe tomatoes as a garnish (in the winter just cherry tomatoes more or less remind you of their taste), so this dish is primarily a summer one. The third indispensable ingredient is *brynza* (feta cheese), it's better to use expensive feta sheep cheese, but it's suitable to use so-called Bulgarian feta cheese, from cows' milk, but only the kind that is sold by weight, pulled out of brine, as it's supposed to be with all brine cheeses. The taste of a hot loaf made of corn flour, salted *brynza* sheep cheese, and fresh tomato combine in a remarkable harmony. They go perfectly with each other – like wood and carpenter's glue, like soft lead and the sharp edges of glass in a classic stained-glass window (please forgive me for the unappetizing nature of my comparisons), like Romeo and Juliet, whom some kind of force tosses into each other's arms (we're speaking here only about the force of interaction).

Thus: take roughly ground corn flour like a light gold semolina (you won't be able to buy Moldovan in Russia, so you'll have to buy Italian "polenta" in supermarkets; don't confuse this kind of flour with a much larger ground grain– you won't get polenta from it, if you only mix it with corn flour, which by appearance is similar to starch; for me it happened that I mixed the leftover "polenta" with grain and flour and achieved results that weren't too bad). Pour it in while you're mixing it into boiling salted water in a proportion of 1:4. After a few minutes it will thicken and begin to bubble up and puff. You'll have to stir it for about twenty minutes. If you add a piece of sweet butter and a few teaspoons of vegetable oil, you don't have to stir it constantly, and you can busy yourself with preparing the remaining ingredients of this dish. That is, you can cut up ripe tomatoes in large pieces, cut up the brynza sheep cheese into large cubes or sticks and spread them out separately on plates or saucers. When during the mixing with a wooden spoon our mamalyga begins to recede from the walls of a deep stewing pan and thickens to such a degree that you can drop it out onto a cutting board and not pour it, do this with a knock

> *– turn over the stewing pan onto the cutting board and with a wide knife or spatula shape the form of a loaf (if there was too little butter and the mamalyga stuck to the bottom). After five minutes you'll be able to cut up the loaf like bread, and lay it out on plates (in its cold form it will lose all its taste and may be useful just for omelets). Three flavors should mix together in your mouth: the steaming mamalyga, the juicy tomato, and salted brynza sheep cheese. Try it – you won't regret it.*

The famous Cossack **kulesh** is close to this dish to a certain degree. It's almost the same light golden color, but only thanks to millet.

> *Millet is cooked for a long time in a large quantity of salted water with a bay leaf. When it becomes similar to thin gruel, you add large cut-up pieces of potato to it (which is a deviation from the canon, but really enriches the taste of the dish) and fried onions and salo (pig lard) or small bits of pork are tossed into a frying pan. Then the pan with the kulesh is covered and stands at low heat until the potatoes are completely ready. This amazingly tasty dish has the same deficiency as polenta-mamalyga. Kulesh in its cold form becomes a shadow of what it was in its freshly prepared hot form.*

Fried Potatoes, Boiled Potatoes...

It's with difficulty that Russia got used to the potato, but once it got used to it–you can't tear it away from it. Only the Belarusians love their potatoes more than the Russians. The Russian classic, of course, is the **soft-boiled light golden potato**. It's fantastic as a stand-alone dish if you flavor it with butter and sprinkle it with dill. Keep in mind that you have to toss the peeled *potatoes* into a small quantity of boiling salted water with bay leaves and boil covered till the first signs of the potatoes becoming soft while the individual potatoes are still whole, but it's already clear that with the slight touch of a fork they'll fall apart. By the way, don't throw away the potato broth – it can be used for cooking a soup or gravy over the course of the next few days.

Boiled potatoes are ideal with pickled *herring* and with onion rings in a lemon-butter sauce. With domestic canned beef, it is very filling and nostalgic. With *pickled cabbage* or *pickled products* as a garnish–it's patriotic.

In the form of a **purée**, boiled potatoes are divinely tender, if you know the main secret of a good purée: you need not just to flavor a purée with butter and add a tablespoon of boiled *milk* a few times, but you also mainly need to whip, whip, whip it, fluff it up to the consistency of a soufflé and eat it hot, that is, right away. Don't be lazy about warming up the plates for the purée–a tender purée on a really large cold plate turns cold instantaneously.

Fried potatoes can be a standalone dish when prepared the right way. The very first condition for proper frying of all ingredients without exception is as follows: they must be as dry as possible and be fried on a well-heated frying pan in hot butter. By the way, you can salt only the butter beforehand, but definitely do not salt the ingredients! In this way, the potatoes are fried with chopped up yellow onions on high heat until they are reddish brown and form a crust–at this stage you need to be right next to the stove. Only after doing this can you significantly lower the heat, add a little more salt to the potatoes, add a few cloves of crushed or finely chopped garlic, cover the frying pan and let the potatoes become soft in the covered pan for about 10 more minutes. You'll have to stir the potatoes a few more times with a spatula, and finally take off the cover for a minute or two for the potatoes to dry out, then turn off the stove and serve it on plates.

Children love **draniki** or **deruny** *(potato pancakes)* more than anything. Grate a peeled potato on a grater–and only on a grater! Keep in mind, by the way, that large young potatoes won't work for potato pancakes because of their high liquid content. On the same grater grate an onion, beat an egg, add salt, and add just a little bit of flour and chopped up dill.

Fry the mixture on hot vegetable oil at medium heat. Flip it over just once. Letting the oil drip off the potato pancakes, stack them on a warmed up and uncovered porcelain plate so that the potato pancakes don't become wet. Eat them piping hot with mildly heated sour cream. You can also eat them with a garnish made of onions with tiny bits of salo (pig lard). You can also eat them with a mushroom-onion sauce. Then you can eat more deruny. In fact there is nothing like potato pancakes.

For a child it's best also to introduce grated squash into the ingredients, from which the deruny taste will become more tender and diet-conscious, and fry it on a non-stick frying pan with just a small amount of butter on low heat.

From the same ingredients as for potato pancakes you can also prepare one big drachena – one really big and fat potato pancake the size of the entire frying pan, a kind of potato sheet cake or **korzh** (*a flat cake*) about an inch and a quarter thick. The drachena is fried on low heat so that it's well cooked. I've invented a way of turning it on the other side. Take a flat plate that's slightly smaller than the frying pan, cover it with vegetable oil and cover the drachena with it on top. Holding the plate with an oven mitt, turn the frying pan upside down. After this return the frying pan onto the burner, and add a little oil or butter to it. When the oil or butter heats up, use a flipper to move the drachena from the plate to the frying pan, cover it with a lid and on low heat prepare it until it's ready. The drachena is cut up like honey-cake and is served covered with sour cream.

Potato shepherd's pie or **zrazy** *is a remarkable dish. Boiled unseasoned ground beef is placed into a small closed pie shell made out of mashed and slightly salted potatoes cooked with their skins on. The top and sides of the casserole are spread with sour cream. The casserole is formed on a baking sheet greased with fat, or in foil greased with sour cream or mayonnaise, into which it's rolled up. In the first instance the casserole will work well with chicken, and in the second it will be steamed and dietary. You can even make the casserole in foil in a roaster in* about ten minutes, but an oven is better. No matter how you cook it, adults and children will like it equally.

Pickled and Marinated Vegetables

Now the season for salting and pickling is coming. It's desirable to do this during the new moon, which sounds unscientific, but is supported by many centuries of practice. All provisions should be fresh, and not kept for long periods of time. The main pickled product of the Russian kitchen is **pickled cabbage**.

Cabbage is pickled in October, after the first frosts hit the cabbage heads (here's something more scientific: in the heads of cabbage something happens with the density and sweetness of the cabbage leaves, and it needs to be accepted on faith as culinary dogma). The best types of cabbage for pickling have a flattened and not an elongated shape. After you remove the upper green leaves, chop the cabbage and grate cleaned carrots on a large grater (in proportions of 15:1), add cranberry (1/2-1/3 times less than the carrots), with your hands press the mixture in an enamel bowl with rock salt (2% of the weight of the cabbage) until the cabbage juice is formed, then tamp with your fists in a large capacity enamel vat, or in a large earthenware jar or small wooden barrel. Spread cabbage leaves over the bottom of the container and set out a layer of medium size Antonov apples (this will be a grand surprise for winter holiday spreads). After completing this step, place the bucket, or whatever you are using, in a warm place – right next to the kitchen stove or next to a radiator, apply pressure (at least using a flat plate beneath a big jar of water), cover it on top with a clean cheesecloth or a linen cloth and once a day push the cabbage to the bottom so that gases can escape. It will release juice, start to foam, and bubble – all these are signs of proper fermentation. Don't let it get chilled – there shouldn't be any drafts or drastic variations in temperature (this pertains to all types of fermentation, whether it be yeast dough or grape wine).

After 5-7 days put it out to a moderately cold place but don't let it freeze (after another month the cold will even be helpful for it, but not earlier). Make sure that the surface of the cabbage is covered with the cheesecloth and cabbage juice – for that you can increase the weight. Don't forget to at least once a week wash the cheesecloth, the plate, or the wooden disk and the weight with hot water in order to avoid the growth of mold.

Now let's turn to **pickled cucumbers**. They should be fresh and of equal size. There is a simple way to force them to become crunchy in pickled form. Simply pour boiling water with rock salt (three full tablespoons per three-liter jar) dissolved in it over the cucumbers. In the jar the cucumbers are interlaid with stalks of dill, a currant leaf, with leaves and slices of horseradish root (to maintain firmness), cherry leaves and celery, along with cleaned whole cloves of garlic. It's also good to use tarragon and sharp red pepper. Thanks to all of this the taste of the properly pickled cucumbers become even richer. A critical moment: before salting and closing the jar shut, it is necessary to sour the pickles, that is, to allow them to ferment for about five days in a warm spot. The brine needs to turn hazy and white. Then you pour it off, boil it, and let it cool to a temperature of 170 degrees Fahrenheit, pour it back, and then hermetically seal the jars (it's most convenient to use screw-down canning jars for this, just make sure the lids are clean and dry). After this take the jars to a cold, dark place.

Pickled tomatoes are such a delight, that they are worth the work you put in to make them. You need to pickle them at the end of August or the beginning of September, while the round and flattened types of tomatoes are still available. They also should be "calibrated" to an average size. Their pickling and salting are very similar to the cucumbers, but you naturally don't pour boiling water over them, but a warm brine (because of the density of the tomato skins you need twice as much salt as for the cucumbers), and they take much longer to pickle. After two days you already can eat a cucumber as a slightly *salted pickle, but a pickled tomato – only after a month. Keep an enamel-lined bucket or small barrel with the tomatoes under pressure in a warm place for at least three weeks, after which you can seal them in glass jars. In addition, boil the brine and pour it over the pickled tomatoes. Their taste is the liveliest if you leave the tomatoes in an open vat weighted down in a cold place. If the process of fermentation has been successful (and here, as with wine, the success is not guaranteed from year to year, a drop in temperature could stop the formation of whitish bubbles of gas under the tomato skin – and this is the top class of pickled tomatoes, there is no better snack for a chaser after drinking vodka, contrary to popular opinion!), then a freezing temperature for them will be like water off a duck's back. Having scraped out from under the crust of ice just such a tomato, you'll be struck by the fact that the freezing even helped it. There's one problem with these pickled tomatoes – they disappear really quickly. Especially if you have children in the house.*

Here it's permissible to make a digression and share a secret for making **sun-dried tomatoes**, not ceding anything to pickled ones in the sense of the development of "tomato dependence." In Western Europe gourmets adore them, but here in Russia they are little known, and at that only in canned form – swimming in olive oil. They reach the peak of taste in a sun-dried form, resembling the consistency of dried apricot, with which everyone is familiar, and in taste – the mysterious quintessence of the very essence of a tomato, not dissimilar to a raw tomato, or tomato juice, but rather – a delicate ritzy cheese. It's so tasty (even children agree) that the need arose to invent a means for drying tomatoes in urban environments.

What you can do anywhere in Italy or in Central Asia right under a killer sun, in Moscow you have to do in an open electric broiler oven, leaving it on overnight at a temperature of 230 degrees F. To achieve this, select ripe tomatoes are cut in half or smaller, sprinkled with rock salt, and placed on a baking sheet.

> *After two or three nights the tomatoes are ready, it just remains to transfer them into a glass jar with a lid and put them in a kitchen cabinet or on a shelf. You can not only snack on them, but the entire winter add them to hot dishes – from borsht to a vegetable-meat ragout (see imam-bayaldy). By the way, in the very same way, just at a lower temperature, you can dry sliced Boletus mushrooms (it is a mystery why they always turn out more fragrant and more tasty than store-bought ones – and this is not just my imagination.*

It's very important not to miss the mushroom season. Marinated Boletus mushrooms with creamy marks on their caps packed in a glass jar are a song, to which only the most unfeeling heart will not respond. But without marinated honey mushrooms you won't be able to prepare complete Russian *shchi* and all kinds of *solyanka*.

> *Pickling them is a breeze: after cleaning the tops and the gills under their caps, wash them well and boil them for about forty minutes in a really large pan or – using the know-how of the Russian villages – simply pour boiling water over them, let them cool off, and repeat the procedure three times. Then marinade them nearly the same way as the cucumbers with herbs and garlic, just without pouring brine over them, but sprinkling the layers with rock salt, place some weight on them, and put them in the refrigerator. After three weeks you can try them and add them to dishes.*

All is clear with marinades, not a word about them – with the exception of a fruit mixture made of peaches and plums in a weak 2-3% acidic marinade and marinated pickles for salad Olivier, but it's easier just to buy them than make them yourself. They know how to marinade at factories, especially sour pickles and gherkins that rarely can be found at outdoor markets in Russia.

It also doesn't hurt to dry a bit of herbs of various types for winter dishes. Best of all – placing them on a clean piece of paper on the hood above the stove. And you need to preserve fresh herbs like this: in a large bunch in a jar with water on the shelf of the refrigerator.

Home-made Fast Food

Fast food can also be surprisingly tasty when it's truly homemade. In the morning it could be common **French toast** made of white bread, well moistened in a whipped egg with milk, lightly salted, and browned on melted butter. They will be a splendid complement to a cup of coffee with milk or cocoa!

It would be even simpler to stick a little piece of French bread on your fork, and brown it on an open gas flame, or warm it in the toaster or on the wire rack of a toaster oven to a crunchy state.

In principle it's a good idea to toast any day-old bread before eating it and freshen dried out bread by tightly wrapping it in aluminum foil and putting it in a toaster oven. Thanks to the remaining moisture in it, it will soften on the tray of the toaster oven in a matter of minutes.

*An **open-faced hot sandwich** will require more effort. On the other hand, by itself it can take the place of a substantial breakfast or lunch. Sprinkle an inch-thick piece of French bread with soy sauce, spread butter on it, place a few pieces of canned Pacific saury or skipper fish on it, cover that with several slices of hard-boiled egg and several slices of fresh cucumber or a pickle, sprinkle with chopped scallions or yellow onions and greens, spread a little bit of mayonnaise and sprinkle with grated cheese, after that place it in the toaster oven for 4-5 minutes. A lot simpler and healthier than this multistoried construction is a hot open-faced sandwich with baloney,[64] covered just with a wedge of pineapple.*

*It's impossible not to say something about a simple dish of **eggs with brisket**, bacon, or even salo (pig lard). First, sauté yellow onions in butter on a frying pan on high heat. To it you add finely chopped brisket and squares of white French bread, (preferably dried to a crunchy state in a toaster oven in advance). After several minutes eggs are added, at least*

---

64 It is called "Doctor's Sausage" in Russian.

one of them should remain sunny-side up. The eggs are salted, sprinkled with chopped green onions and greens, and if you desire – with grated cheese. Do not cover the eggs with a lid, and do not over-dry them, work it a little bit with a spatula. Serve it hot, steaming and with a wafting aroma.

When I stay up too late, I sometimes prepare these kinds of eggs even at night, which is awfully unhealthy, but devilishly tasty. My sleepy wife sometimes comes out at the scent and sounds reaching her from the kitchen, and then, of course, I'm obliged to share it with her.

A dietary **steamed omelet**, which is extremely easy to prepare, will be better for children and the elderly. Pour a glass or two of water into a pot and bring it to a slow boil. In a large tea bowl, well greased with butter, whip an egg until it turns frothy, and salt it. Stirring it, add a little bit of sifted flower, and place the tea bowl into the pot. Cover the tea bowl with a saucer, and the pot – with a cover, and keep it on the burner for ten minutes. You'll end up with the tenderest airy omelet that you need to eat immediately before it sags in (for it not to sag, you can add a pinch of baking soda, though the taste of the omelet will become more coarse).

And finally, the Soviet classic – **navy-style macaroni.** Somehow people are getting too lazy to prepare it, but boiled meat is almost always left in the refrigerator from bouillon. You need to grind it through a meat grinder. In a frying pan sauté onions with vegetable oil, add boiled ground meat, a little bit of chopped greens, and boiled macaroni (the best of them are those requiring the longest cooking time – for cooking time look at the instructions on the package; cook them in a large quantity of salted boiling water with bay leaves), then combine all the ingredients, cover the dish with a pot cover and for a few minutes keep it on a stove with the burner turned off. Pickles go very well with this dish. The dish is an unsophisticated one, but very solid and filling.

PART IV
Cities and Dishes

Hamburg and Munich

From the story "Zimania. Germa"[65] *(Wintgerm. Gerwint)*

Lobster and Others

At every step in Germany and in German-speaking Switzerland you can hear: "Tschüs" – meaning "Bye, all the best, I am gone," which, to your untrained ear, sounds like the English word "Cheese," so you rush immediately to buy it, and not just it: you eat it, keep eating it, and keep on eating it!

They say that the majority of Russian visitors are indifferent and often simply have no feeling for the huge world of gustatory sensation that is revealed to them – their chores seem to be more important. I doubt that the Russian world is anti-hedonistic in principle. The answer is, rather, that those who come from Russia represent a specific type of intellectuals, who spend so much time talking at the kitchen table that one of their senses atrophied in the process of historical development; their tongues have become encrusted with a deposit of ideas, notions, and calories that block out their gustatory receptors. That is most likely the reason why the inhabitants of the Old World become so surprised and animated when they meet a different type of a Russian who is interested in the taste of what he eats, and they rush to acquaint him with all the new foods, delicacies, and gustatory sensations that, in their opinion, deserve special attention.

Properly speaking, the German kitchen does not represent anything special, with the exception of light beer and different types of hams. Nowhere else in the world as in Germany can breathtaking gherkins be spoiled with vinegar, can the taste of common mayonnaise and mustard be destroyed with aromas and sweeteners, and can the taste of herring be stifled with apples and sour cream; all

---

65 In the original Russian text Klekh plays with words "Germaniia" (Germany) and "zima" (winter), out of which he forms two neologisms: "Zimaniia" and "germa."

these cause unbearable suffering among emigrants from *Russland* and Ukraine, they exude poisonous saliva that damages their stomachs.

However, thank God, thanks to the expansion of the Italians, Turks, Greeks, and, not to a small degree, to the books of Elizabeth David[66] and those of other authors, a wave of Mediterranean cuisine is washing over Europe. I am not even speaking here about the invisible presence and influence of the great French gastronomic empire, as well as of the offerings of the select best of everything that is caught and grows all over the world... Lobsters and oysters, Parmesan and Gorgonzola cheeses, smoked salmon and grilled giant shrimps, octopi, ravioli-al-pasta, the "salmon's dialogue" with something else – I don't remember – and tartlet with "caviar," broccoli cream soup and fried zucchini, pickled artichokes, Kirsch brandy fondue with croutons and Tiramisu (which you have to eat with your eyes closed), espresso and cappuccino, Italian ice cream with Grand Marnier liqueur (which is the best in the world), marzipans and salted pistachios, and avocados that are like spring water – these are nothing but the Great Gastronomic Adventure that unexpectedly fell as an avalanche onto us as a reminder of the formidable beauty of the world.

How can you believe that Italians can poison a Russian person?

After my editor and I, barely restraining ourselves from indecent moaning, tried ravioli in basil and garlic sauce in a small Italian restaurant, I suddenly understood, with all my essence, with my entire stomach, and with spasms in my alimentary canal, something about the reason for Gogol remaining in Rome,[67] about his persistent feeding of the Aksakovs[68] with Italian food, about

---

66 Elizabeth David (1913-1992) was a popular British writer on European cuisine. In the 1950s-1970s she authored several books on Mediterranean, French, Italian, and British cuisine. She was recipient of several prestigious English and French awards, including the 1982 Royal Society of Literature award.

67 Gogol spent 12 years in Italy, which was reflected in several of his later writings.

68 Sergey and Ivan Aksakov were prominent men of letters in Russia in the middle of the 19th century and the major representatives of the Slavophile movement in Russia.

Gogol's deathbed fasting,[69] and why his confessor Father Matvey Konstantinovsky had eaten some kind of sticky muck scooped from the bottom of an opened grave in Torzhok, dirt that turned out to be curative for him, and of course I could not help but remember Pushkin's last communion – his last "good bye" to this world – his brilliant infused fen-berries.[70]

... On one of the first days of my stay at a villa in Altona, I lugged home my long-awaited lobster. Half of the reason for getting it consisted of philology: lobster in Russia is *"omar"*... Homer, in German it is *Hummer*; my hostess Frau Luisa suddenly became agitated, my action reminded her something of the grand style of the past when she was the wife of a Geschäftsführer and used to vacation in Hawaii. She asked me: "Igorrr, and how are you going to cook it?" "Cook it? What do you recommend, Frau Luisa," I found a quick answer. "You know, I'd suggest you prepare it American style." "Wonderful. Let's cook it together and eat it."

My help was not needed in this undertaking; all I had to do was to watch. After throwing the lobster into salted boiling water for two minutes and, at the same time, melting garlic butter with spices in a frying pan, she plopped the lobster on a large dish, sprinkled it with squeezed lemon, and brought it to a small round table that she had set up in the library by a huge window overlooking the Elbe and the evening port.

"What would you like to drink with the lobster?" She asked next. "Drink? Here, I brought two bottles of good dark beer." I had specially looked for it, although the villa's cellars had an endless amount of light beer along with white and red wines. German wines,

---

69 During the last weeks before his death in 1852, Gogol, who all his life was obsessed with food, decided to fast before Maslenitsa (the week-long feast before the beginning of Lent), but was unable to do so. The mental and physical strain led to a sharp deterioration in his condition. Treatment with leeches prescribed by doctors failed, and Gogol died at the age of 42.

70 It is a well-known fact that during last days of his life, when he was lying severely wounded in his apartment in St. Petersburg, Pushkin asked for the infused fen-berries to quench his thirst. He developed a taste for infused fruit and berries during his exile in 1830 in the village of Mikhailovskoe.

though, leave a lot to be desired, rarely are any of them very good. "Igorrr," Frau Louisa said, becoming serious all of sudden, "you won't get a sense of the taste of lobster with that!" And she added resolutely: "You know, I have a couple of bottles of champagne somewhere. I'll be right back." After standing up, she flew up to the second floor like a little girl and brought back four little bottles (each not more than a glass) of champagne.

"Oh, it's beautiful!" She kept saying in English every time she put a piece of lobster, sprinkled with lemon and dipped in hot garlic butter, into her mouth, chasing it with the champagne, nodding her head, and closing her eyes. "It iz nice evening," she kept saying in English in a drawn-out manner. We shared a limited number of English words between us. It was truly a "lovely evening," and it was a miracle that I avoided the temptation not to sense the taste of the lobster and gobble it up, like a slob, as if it were a coarsely tasting crayfish, and chasing it with port wine. Maybe that too wouldn't have been too bad.

My hostess told me that evening after refusing coffee and desert because few people in Germany risk drinking coffee after 2:00 P.M.: "I'm terribly afraid of sharks." I sat deeper in the armchair, lit my cigarette, and proudly answered her: "In our country no one is afraid of sharks."

The Munich Strategy

Wines are another topic.

Winter, what should we do in Germany? Drink, of course, my friend Virgil. Should I order the horse be hooked up to the cart?

Blessed is one who has a guide in the world of libations and cities, as you do in Munich, because cities are not this and that as the Greek philosopher said, but the people who live in them.

The same evening after I had made a devastating raid on a French cellar and filled my flasks with wine from a barrel, tasting it and discussing it with the proprietor; and then, having gathered up as many bottles as my hands could hold, I dragged them to a meat pie dinner with my compatriots and from there, having confused everything and everybody by the end of the evening and gotten a sourness in my mouth from the infectious discussion of politics that accumulated in the pores of the skin, hair, under my nails, and the seams of my clothes, my friend and I made a series of devastating raids at Munich pubs, catching them unaware. We did not stay very long in any one of them, leaving them without any regrets and going to new ones, until in one of them we walked into "The Cyclops," the twelfth chapter of Joyce's *Ulysses* where a tall, cleanly shaven German with pursed lips, pretending to be garrulous, got me to talk over a huge mug of young hoppy beer in order to work up a head of steam: "Aha! An anticommunisto! A spiono! German money!" "What kind of craziness is this?" And, understanding just every other word, I responded with my own attack, and he, having understood that after all there were two of us, he sat down and then moved away, continuing to mutter something under his breath. But this effervescent life is not given to you for arguing in a pub with someone who feels eternally bypassed by it. We went to several other *Kneipes* until the quietly fallen snow revealed the disappearance of a bowler hat for one of us and the absence of a cigarette holder in my pocket. You must drink in establishments and areas that you know. We popped in several pubs that by then were about to close, weaving our way through the empty midnight streets – it was all in vain and was the same as looking for a needle in a haystack. The cigarette holder would be found the next morning; I had already learned its foul habit of disappearing, so that the next morning, conspiring with pangs of conscience, I felt like I have a nail in my head. But the bowler hat – alas! Ah, what a bowler hat it was! What wondrous heavenly hat maker molded you according to a model created by a master's hand? The face of your friend was pressed in it like a red beet in a deep bowl. One day before the hat's disappearance, in the hallways of the "Radio Liberty" station we witnessed a small commotion that grew into real pandemonium in the lobby. Invalids dropped their crutches, hurrying to touch my friend even as they were falling. "May I stand next to you?" "Can you wait a minute, I want my wife to see you." "Would it be too much to ask you to wear the bowler hat tomorrow, I want to take a picture with you." Invitations and requests were fired one after another. Why did all these people become so agitated? In West Berlin I saw a man walking wearing a top hat and white scarf and another one who stepped outside to have a smoke and pass gas.

"I've found my cigarette holder, and you're nothing but a sad sack!" I said to my friend a day later – deliberately rudely, trying to drive away the last remnants of the mercilessly suppressed uprising of my conscience. "I'm a sad sack because I forgot to hide the first volume of Fabre's *Life of Insects*.[71] I knew that when a fellow writer comes to visit, I need to hide everything!" He answered, sincerely lamenting the loss.

A few weeks later he would add to that, speaking with me on the phone: "I brought home a different hat from London, no, not a bowler hat. I dedicate that ill-fated bowler hat to you!"

The quiet city street, which was seemingly brought overnight to Munich from Dikanka,[72] was covered by the lightest, definitely manufactured-by-the-heavens snow. On Saturday morning the sun came out, and my friend the guide and I set out, knee-deep in this blinding down, along this blessed mixture of heaven and hell, in the direction of the Viktualienmarkt, because in Munich you just go there to sober up – with oysters and white wine. The small square in the very center of Munich – the market proper – nearly exactly resembled the Stanislavsky Market[73] in the late 1950s – early 1960s for me: similar low-roofed pavilions, stalls, and kiosks, surrounded by three- or four-storied buildings of the late 19th century. The only difference consisted in the fact that in Munich everything tasty and

---

71 Jean-Henri Casimir Fabre (1823 - 11, 1915) was a French entomologist and author, best known for his studies of insects, and is considered by many to be the father of modern entomology.

72 A reference to Nikolai Gogol's first book of Ukrainian-themed stories *Evenings on a Farm near Dikanka*, in which Gogol tells of magical happenings in the small village of Dikanka on Christmas Eve.

73 Stanislav or Stanislaviv is the old name for the city in Western Ukraine that is now called Ivano-Frankivsk.

edible in the world was here: sea crayfish crawled in the aquariums, 400-kilogram tuna swam in the pools, fruit and vegetable bins contained, along with some familiar specimens, strange fruits and forms of nature; acres of stone pavement were covered with wine crates. In them, interlaid with wood shavings, there were bottles of French, Italian, and Spanish wines. An old man in a light coat and fur hat with a visor played the street-organ with gusto, putting all his body into it and stamping his foot.

For half a day after that I couldn't wash away or swallow the taste of oysters that got stuck in my nose and throat – indissoluble and primordial, like the taste of a popsicle that you suck on in your childhood or matzo bread. As my guide expressed the sensation rather precisely: "It was as if a sea grotto had opened in your mouth." It wasn't just the sea salt, and not the snivel of the first, always unexpected tide of a head cold, it was something else. It is simply the fact that common oysters with their genially blank taste, like an outstanding actor, can absorb and express anything – like that morning, for example.

Berlin, Germany

From the story "Crocodiles Don't Dream"

A certain persistent odor emanated from this barbarian who had arrived from the East. The odor was definitely human, one can even say – masculine, but people should not be so odiferous; it is really too much. After all, there are certain remedies for that.

The food, which this man whom the host had let in his house was cooking, also had the same irritatingly aggressive character. The cat was the first to betray her master. She didn't leave the foreigner's side and rubbed herself against his legs while he cooked and fried something on several burners at the same time, without sparing onion, garlic, spices, and some sauces in microscopic bottles that he had bought. You couldn't say he was making himself feel at home in that apartment or behaving discourteously, but in him there wasn't even any slightly apologetic attitude or any sense of dependence. They were absent not only in his free-wheeling movement through the space of the three-story apartment in which he lived on the third floor, but also in the short conversations that his landlord from time to time started with him in poor English, which neither of them had mastered. Often the threads of a conversation would get hung up and broken, running into a collision with a completely forgotten word; the threads had to be cut and later tied with small knots through strong gesticulation. English was a neutral middle ground between the owner of the apartment and his temporary tenant, and the host was uncomfortable feeling himself almost equal with this man who had come here even without house slippers and who looked perplexed in the simplest of situations; but there was apparently little embarrassment about it as if he and his host had come out onto ice without skates. It was also unpleasant to the host that some things about which his tenant wasn't supposed to have heard FROM BEYOND THE WALL turned out to be not only known to him, but he also commented on them as though he were on friendly terms with them, as though these things were his close friends.

The cat started to turn her nose away from the tin cans with her feline face carnivorously licking her lips on the label and, demonstratively bolting through her cat door in the large door, departed into the garden. The host's first-grade daughter started to look in disgust at the ready-made food, sealed in plastic that was offered to her, and with a fork she grudgingly poked at the boxed food of who knows what, something she had tired of even before she had been born, and kept glancing time and again at what was being cooked in the kitchen. During one of the first few days while the tenant was living there, both the father and his daughter ate up a bowl each of a simple soup cooked with vegetables in intoxicatingly pungent broth with cauliflower that resembled granular caviar that ends up stuck between your teeth. From that moment on the father apparently decided on behalf of both of them to refuse to eat the offerings that he saw as incursions of disturbing, suspicious, and, certainly, an unhealthy kitchen. For example, the tenant drank tea with lemon, cut them into neat disks, in huge quantities, and with great relish his host advised him not to do it because everyone knew that lemon is good only for extracting juice from it, since its skin is sprayed with all kinds of poison, which his foreigner had dissolved in the boiled water. The tenant readily believed him. He had a certain lightness about him, a certain illusively perverse lightness. He was the first person "from there" whom the host had seen up close; he was a son of those people against whom his father had been fighting.

Mr. Epsilon the tenant suddenly also developed problems with acclimatization. It turned out that the biting remark has an inverse effect as well: what for a Russian is death is good for a German. Last time he was in this country, the tenant traveled mostly on field rations and didn't pay much attention to it. All products had only a nominally approximate resemblance to those he used in his life. He had to exert great efforts to find decent vinegar or sour cream that would be the real thing. Even the most ordinary cabbage desperately resisted his effort to incorporate it into soup and remain firm without losing its consistency and falling to the bottom of the pot.

Lucerne, Switzerland

From the essay "A Month in Switzerland"

I was the first Russian in the Haus-am-See Hotel near Lucerne (with deviant behavior at that – as for the Swiss so for the Swiss Russians), and many were intrigued by the "Rusisch Schriftschteller" from Moscow. Undoubtedly, the matter wasn't about me, but about the reputation that Russian literature has gained in the world, about the immense size of the world called Russia, and, finally, about Moscow, which all of Switzerland would not be enough to populate and the diameter of which is equal the distance from Zurich to Lucerne – just imagining this would terrify you! I was observed and even tested a few times – what do I think about what happened to the NTV channel?[74] Do I

---

74 A reference to the events in May 2000 when the police stormed the headquarters of the NTV station and Media Most company owned by the oligarch Vladimir Gusinsky, who was critical of Putin's policies and the second Chechnya war. Gusinsky was arrested and later released but forced to immigrate to Israel. The NTV and Media

like money the way a wild boar loves – dirt? And the most intimate question – was I capable of appreciating the merits of the *Underwalden* cuisine that many have disputed?

My God, it was the first time that I ate so well in Switzerland! I didn't hold back my carnivorous moan in a small Sarnen restaurant (where two Lucerne patriots had brought me) when I put the first piece of the signature dish of one of the four "forest cantons" (the original ones – from "where the Swiss land is and came to be"). The dish was Bratwurst with Zwiebelsauce and Rienschleims – fried pork garlic kielbasa with onion sauce and undercooked potato flapjacks that tasted heavenly after all that healthy and nutritious cosmopolitan nonsense with little difference in taste and smell!

The water in Lake Vierwaldstättersee (Lake Lucerne) on the shore of which I lived for a month is so clean that fish don't live in it – there's nothing to eat for them, and the fishermen who keep pulling out empty nets in all the lake's coves, I think, are hired by tourist companies to create a picturesque impression. You could see with your naked eye they were nothing else but pretenders. I had some illegal homemade fishing tackle with me. (What other tackle could I have? I couldn't enroll in and successfully pass some "fishing course" in order to get a license that would allow me to fish in a Swiss reservoir that, as it turned out, had no fish). However, after I watched the hard and futile labor of the Swiss fishermen and admired the transparency of the water (you could see the fishing line in the water even from NATO fighter planes that were flying overhead, and the fish, if they were there, could look straight into a fisherman's eyes reproachfully nodding their heads; I didn't even dare test my homemade tackle for bottom fishing, this brainchild of a lazy Russian "lefthander," in these neutral waters.

I saw Vierwaldstättersee trout only in fishing guides; it is difficult to buy it even at the Saturday market at the Lake Lucerne embankment, which has whatever you might be looking for. But if you don't have fish, you don't have seagulls. The birds here, unlike

---

Most were acquired by Gazprom and fell under government control.

those on Lake Zurich, are all either black or spotted, only swans are white. If you hear double-leafed doors slamming on the water, it means that a swan, having stretched its snake-like neck, is running the 100-meter distance along the water in order once again to shame the laws of Newton's physics and, having lifted its fat, heavy bottom from the surface of the water, to take a slow contoured flight to a more satisfying cove. And some devil cried out during the night, calling or trying to frighten me: "Oo-oo-oo! Oo-goo-go-go!" One night I found it and recorded its voice – it turned out to be some horned owl, a Waldkauz. Several of them took a fancy to the tops of the sequoias that were planted a hundred years ago on the shore of the lake, from which the owls called to one other before starting their nocturnal mouse hunt. The Swiss call the sequoia a mammoth tree. This name immediately brings to mind the mural in the Lucerne Gletschergarten "The View of Lucerne 16 Thousand Years Ago," in which a couple of mammoths gaze on the plateau from some elevation, observing how the glaciers, snaking and crumbling, crawl to devour the plateau. When the glaciers retreated, the mammoths disappeared, and the city was built on this spot.

I was totally baffled by the sex life of clams in green shells. After I spread the delicacy on a dish and unfolded the indecent mantles of the shell-fish, I discovered to my amazement that a part of them grew some small dark brown members, which in disgust I tore out by the root and only after that started my meal. They must have become bored living on the bottom and in the darkness of their closed shucks, and because of that, they've developed their bi-sexuality. Other than that they were very tasty with a tinge of the hardboiled yellow of an egg, an exciting dish it was.

Loneliness disposes one to the development of sensuality. I even attempted to prepare an artichoke, but wasn't able to make its rough petals soft, no matter how hard I tried. I had to take it apart and suck the flesh off them after dipping them in a sauce and throwing the rest away when I finished. My Swiss acquaintances, who at some time in the past had tried to prepare artichoke, were making merry at my expense with great satisfaction. They're culinary chauvinists!

Sea crayfish are another matter, that *salo* (pig lard) of the seas, capable of competing with smoked salmon for the tenderest salt pickling. While its flesh was melting in my mouth, being washed down into my stomach by a foamy wave of beer (I didn't provide myself with a chilled white wine), I understood why the largest whales eat plankton – because, most likely, there is nothing tastier than plankton in the whole wide world. With their size they could snack on any other living creature, but they choose krill and plankton – nutritious bouillon without bones, which readily floats into your mouth on its own; all you have to do is to drop your lower jaw. What pleasure-seekers they are! (I want to think that they are kind creatures because of their size, like the grass-eating elephants that are relatively peaceful and fearful only of tamers and evil mice that gnaw holes in their soft soles – as everyone knows, elephants walk on tiptoes.

I remember my jaws contracting when for the first time I sank my teeth into a solid piece of Parmesan cheese, more than anything its flaky consistency, scent, and appearance resembled a callus – it turned out to be so tasty! Each gourmet has his winning place in every category. I would place cheeses in the following order: the first place would belong to the French Roquefort-type cheeses, the second – to the Italian chunk (never grated under any circumstances!) Parmesan, the third – to Swiss Gruyère, and the complimentary bronze medal would be divided by the Swiss Emmentaller and the Hutsul[75] goat-cheese feta. I would not allow the most popular among domestic cheese-eaters, the sluggish and tasteless "Rossiisky" (Russian) cheese, to take part in the competition at all.

However, tastes change, everyone knows that. But there is one small problem here: the kitchen is a rightful and integral element of cultures. If you see Hegel in the philosophy of a particular culture, then you'll see Bach and Beethoven in music (and no sitar!) and

---

75 Hutsuls are mountain people, who live in the Carpathian Mountains in Western Ukraine.

will eat sausages and drink beer. If, to the contrary, you have the sitar in music, then you'll chew on some vegetable stalks and eat curried rice. Etc.

So I wonder now if I'm not a true Catholic? Or perhaps a supporter of Ecumenism and a shameful eclectic. As soon as I return home, I'll first of all demand the "stewed" cabbage *shchi* soup with pickled honey mushrooms and sour cream, soft-boiled potatoes with butter and piquant pickled herring, and I cook scorching hot Ukrainian red borsht. Here in Switzerland I'm a guest and have no time to do it. I eat what I'm given or what I accidently or out of curiosity come across in order not to be distracted, so that my brain works in an efficient manner.

There were a few small things left to be taken care of: the move to the St. Niklausen Hotel (the "Ordnung" faltered, the mistake had been input in it from the beginning), farewell dinners, suppers, and strolls. Then there was Lucerne and the morning train straight to Zurich Airport. From there my bag with the manuscript, a month's worth of writing, would set out to Muslim Tunis, but the latter would disgorge it (perhaps because of the last piece of the Ukrainian *salo* left with me by a former acquaintance from Lviv, who was visiting me in Lucerne – I felt bad about throwing the *salo* out – and an opened bottle of Montepulciano, my great thanks to them for that), and on the third after my return, the lost and found service of Sheremetevo Airport would deliver the unlucky traveler straight to my house in the Yasenovo district in Moscow where my wife and I were renting an apartment. It's true: all's well that ends well.

In Switzerland I was writing a novella about life in a vanished country, which occupies one sixth of the world's landmass. Now, sitting in Moscow, I was writing about Switzerland – about the vision of Mt. Rigi and life on the shore of the lake. Although, perhaps, it only seemed to me that I was writing about Switzerland, and I was writing about myself or about Russia or for Russia, and also for Galicia (which somehow became a second homeland for me), for former inhabitants of Lviv, and for citizens of the vanished countries, I am writing about something as distant and abstract for them as life on Mars.

Aqaba, Jordan

From the essay "Jordan – from Friday to Friday"

The less than an hour travel time from the waterless Bedouin desert to the shore of the caressing sea was a big and, I won't conceal it, pleasant surprise. First of all I want to sing the praise of the Jordanian roads – they are wonderful (built with Iraqi money during the Iran-Iraq war when Iraq received the lion's share of imports through Jordan's Aqaba. I didn't see them being repaired anywhere (although in the rest of the world, that is, the permanent condition of roads); that means the local climate is their friend, not an enemy. Secondly, the nasty looking mountain range as though it were a clay mass piled up effectively by a bulldozer from three sides covers Jordan's Aqaba and Israel's Eilat – two parts of a settlement that used to be called Ailat. Because of this mountain ridge, Aqaba has a unique greenhouse microclimate and eternal summer. Thirdly, a seaport is always a gateway to the wide world. This is the place where Jordan delivers its phosphates via the narrow gauge Hedjaz railway and delivers potash by trucks from the Al-Lisan Peninsula on the Dead Sea, and from here drives cisterns with crude oil for producing gas, etc. to the north.

To stimulate trade, Aqaba was made a free economic zone. As a result of that, you can find beer (on the level of the Soviet "Zhiguli" brand), 100-proof anise arrack (everything is aromatized here – coffee with cardamom, tea with mint, etc.), and inexpensive wine (on which I decided not to waste my time) as much as you wish any time of the day. This small town is as close as you can have to western standards. These kinds of commercial districts can be found in an ethnic area of any of the European capitals. It's pleasant to meet your acquaintances – Souffian or Mahmoud here and have tea right there on the spot in a store.

By the way, tea is the hottest thing served in Jordan. After all, what can desert dwellers know of culinary art and gastronomy? The Jordanian kitchen is being Americanized by leaps and bounds – all these little trays with tasteless salads, pseudo-shishkebab, and several characterless national dishes. The only worthwhile dishes are freshly baked bread, freshly squeezed lemon juice, hummus, and white eggplant caviar. Only in Aqaba have restaurants preserved their distinct face – there you can eat sea perch and drink strong coffee nearly without the cardamom.

Lastly, the sea completely won my heart. It was exactly as I said – caressing, as though baking powder and vinegar were dissolved in water so your hair would be fluffy. There is also coral somewhere, but I didn't see it at the beach of the Movenpick Hotel, a twin of the one that remained on the shore of the Dead Sea. There wasn't a clay village here, but there were many more water attractions, including a sauna, Jacuzzi pools, a beach with a pier, and various sea creatures. I also remember a guard wearing a sweater early in the morning and with a mixture of compassion and disgust looking at this swimmer coming out of the water. The water temperature was not less than 20°C, the day before it was 25°C, after all it was December. Only the most daredevil and miscreant Muslims appreciate bathing in the sea (not to speak of Muslim women bathing in the sea, for them it is taboo). I felt fantastic!

After haggling, Sergei bought an "ancient" metal mug that turned out to be "Made in Germany;" I – a small toy camel with little bells on its neck and a zipper on its belly for my daughter; and Nikolai – a candlestick with a shade that will remind him of the Wadi Rum Desert. Even Sufian bought some trinket on the boardwalk of Aqaba that was ten times cheaper there. I think now that the only good buy for all of us would have been prayer beads, so that we could finger them now while sitting in the snowy Moscow, Amman, or Bryansk forest where Nikolai lives, taking a walk down memory lane and rolling the names of the places we visited off our tongues: Amman, Jerash, Madaba, Mt. Nebo, Bethany, Mudjib, Karak, Petra, Wadi Rum, Aqaba, Amman – Moscow.

Tomso, Norway

From the sketch "The Norwegian Subarctic"

I can't be silent about my impression of the city of Tomso, which is called "the little Paris" of Northern Norway. In my opinion, by its scale and landscape, it reminds me more of Swiss Lucerne and by its planning and buildings – an American university town in Massachusetts or Pennsylvania, especially taking into consideration the fact that ten thousand out of the seventy-five thousand of its population consist of students.

The city is old and new, lively and very beautiful, even at night. In its port a snow-white cruise ship sits next to a three-mast sailboat, a cargo ship – next to a motorized ocean yacht. Bridges connect islands to the continental part of the city; a cable lift stretches from the bank of a fjord to a restaurant on top of a mountain; the triangular Arctic Cathedral (which is also called the "Cathedral of the Arctic Ocean") resembles an ice mound. It was the city where Amundsen prepared and equipped his polar expeditions. One of the rooms in the inn where he always stayed has its walls covered with photographs of those expeditions, and the restaurant is famous for its French-Norwegian cuisine.

No one can forget the pungent taste of the Kamchatka crab soup and the tender consistency of the roasted venison, stewed to the consistency of boiled cow tongue in a quick-cooker and served with white Alsace or Australian red wine, or a raisin desert wine. The feast is the celebration of the belly's name day[76] and the return to civilization.

The city of Tromso has a double debt to Russia, and many here remember it. The first is that the city was founded on this wild shore thanks to Russian coast-dwellers, who, at the beginning of the 18th century, started to sail there and trade without paying customs taxes. By the end of the 18th century the Norwegian authorities lost their

---

76 In Soviet times there was no distinction made between a saint's name day and one's birthday.

patience and built a customs office here with which the city had begun. The second debt is that during WWII the city was saved by Soviet troops from destruction. The retreating German divisions burned Northern Norwegian cities and towns such as Alta and Budo to the ground, but they did not have time to do it to Tromso.

Vilnius, Lithuania

From the essay "Free Vilnius"

Is It Easy to Get Lost in Vilnius?

Lithuania already begins when you get on the train "Moscow-Vilnius," which is extremely clean, with deodorizers in the restrooms, and starched bedding that departs from the Belarusian Train Station. It's true that in the morning the curious and distrustful border guards would take your luggage apart, looking in every nook and cranny, but you can understand them – Soviet power is still in Gudogay on the Belarusian side, and at the neighboring station Kena in Lithuania, there is a Scandinavian style train station and next to the Lithuanian flag, a starry banner of the European Union flutters in the wind. The border was real, as it used to be, with an endless electric fence along the tracks and video cameras. I unwittingly thought that Lithuanians with their new friends had built another "Kaliningrad corridor" for us, but fortunately all these "VOKHR" (armed guard) delights ended after a dozen kilometers. A half hour later we arrived in Vilnius, fresh after a good night's sleep, and bathing in the morning sun.

I exchanged Euros for *litai* (there *litai* were still used, although with a Lithuanian passport you could travel through all Western Europe without worrying about visas). It's better not to bring rubles here. The ruble exchange rate for the *litai* is approximately 10:1, but in the majority of currency exchanges they buy it from you for 7 cents and sell it for 14. Nothing like that happens to any other currency, and this was the only expression of the "Russophobia" that I encountered in the five days that I spent there, if we don't take into consideration the fact that the train speaker system said good-bye to the passengers in Lithuanian and English; apparently all the Russians had gotten off along the way and the train had filled up with a hell of a lot of Englishmen.

I have to say from the start that Vilnius pleasantly surprised me and dispelled the bad feeling I had when I was there in the late 1980s. At that time it looked excessively politicized, uptight and flat, as though nothing but squares and sidewalks were left in it, and all the walls were gone. To be objective, many other cities looked exactly like that – bare, but each had its own fate and destiny. The Lithuanian capital after ten years has finally regained its History, which rushed like blood to its anemic cheeks.

I strolled along the central Gediminas Prospect, enjoying the sun and coolness in the ancient city, which was just waking up. It was later that I "disqualified" this street: why did they cut down the old shady linden trees, leaving just cast iron fences on the sidewalks? Why did they sterilize and stylize this street after some average and no one's "European city," while the entire charm of Vilnius lies in something else? The present and future of Vilnius greatly depends on developing international tourism. Simple-minded people think that to do it they must shampoo the city, apply perfumed deodorizers to it, and slick it into oblivion in the German style. That is why you should visit Vilnius now while that has not yet happened. The city is worth it. Three days are enough for a stroll through the city, five if you want to include its environs, but if you want to spend time on the beach or in the countryside, then you will need anything between a week and a month. It cannot be longer than that – you risk becoming a Lithuanian, besides, your visa will not allow it.

"You have a five-day visa, don't be late," a Lithuanian customs officer "graciously" told me while stamping my passport.

I answered in indignation: "I have a return ticket!"

What is the secret of attraction and charm of the Lithuanian capital for the countless crowds of visiting Poles (while you have quite enough of those who live here), for not very wealthy Germans, many English and Americans, and now even for Japanese and St. Petersburgers? The answer most likely lies in the fact that Vilnius is multi-faceted, polyphonic, and multi-dimensional. It could also be the unique contrast between a well-tended and untended view of the city – their mixture and alternation are very refreshing.

The population of Vilnius is well disposed toward tourists and no longer frightens the latter with their mass protest demonstrations. What would they live on if they did not have the transit of goods (legal and illegal) between Western Europe and Russia and tourism? Nowadays only one-third of the products produced in Lithuania reaches the standards of the European Union, and even this is done with difficulty. Lithuanians themselves now are in no hurry to close the damned Ignalina Nuclear Power Plant, trying to figure out how to prolong its life (and it is also somewhat of an honor to have a nuclear power plan, not everyone has one). The other thing is – the gasoline prices keep going up, and all of Lithuania drives slightly used or totally new foreign cars. Just imagine this contrast: a crimson Ferrari is driven into a grass-covered Vilnius yard with crooked barns – right out of a movie set!

Vilnius has five-star hotels, national ethnic restaurants, cafes, and beer bars for any taste; here and there they even serve game, and the service is quite good. But if you set out for a stroll, without fail you will come across blank walls with paint peeling, spacious monastery cloisters and enclosed flower gardens, or tidied-up ruins. Cramped streets draw you in, they break and begin to bend in all directions: up and down, right and left. For the sake of making it unassailable, the Grand Duke Gediminas founded his new Lithuanian capital, on these hills between two rivers after almost seven centuries ago after he had a dream about an iron wolf. In the Köln Atlas of European cities published two hundred years later, Vilnius' city blocks look quite regular. Perhaps later, the Jewish artisans, merchants, and rabbis muddled things up. I'm an experienced traveler and "draw" plans of cities almost immediately in my head. It's easy to imagine then how delighted I was when by the end of the first day after our long stroll through the old city (without knowing where I was going – wherever our feet and our free mind would take me[77]), I suddenly realized that... I was lost. The city twisted and turned me like a billiard ball, it played me as though it was alive. I think that is why people flock to cities like Vilnius. For a short time they escape the world in which everything has become familiar ad nauseam so that, finding themselves in an unfamiliar place, they just like to take a stroll through a city, as if it had been created specially for walking.

And if you want a snack, you can go almost anywhere, although Lithuanian cuisine is basically a peasant one and is really nothing special in the culinary sense. The old Lithuanian beer soup with sour cream is quite interesting. Western Lithuanian lumberjacks horribly reeked of it. The Belarusian-Polish influence gave birth to the Lithuanian "zeppelins" made out of shredded potatoes with meat filling, and the Crimean-Turkic – "*koldunais*," Lithuanian dumplings with meat and mushroom filling. Nowadays you can be served Ukrainian borsht, Georgian shish kebab, sushi, and, if you look for it, bear meat.

The present artful balance of conveniences and ruin will last for no more than twenty years, but the Lithuanians themselves grossly exaggerate the rumors of the astronomical costliness of life after joining the European Union.

Riga, Latvia

From the essay "Riga Today and Forever"

Gates and the Belly of Riga

I was pleasantly surprised with Riga's train station. Externally the building has not changed, but the Rigans gutted it, opened it up, and brought the interiors to European standards. It became clean, spacious and functional. The square in front of the station has

---

[77] A reference to A. Pushkin's poem "To the Poet" (1830).

been transformed as well – here the god of trade Mercury dealt his magic, having placed glass cubes and towers all along the square's perimeter, ugly if you compare them to the buildings of Old Riga and beautiful if you compare them to the structures from Soviet times – it depends how you look at them. In order not to return to this southern part of the city, it is worth mentioning several of its sights and dominant factors. The peeling "Stalin skyscraper," a reduced-in-size copy of those in Moscow, and an unusual, three-legged TV tower on the other side of the river that you can see from afar. Lithuania's largest (two-story) Russian bookstore "The Mountain" was opened near the skyscraper, which houses the local Academy of Sciences. Not all Rigans know about it yet, but they will have something to read.

However, the most amazing place in this part of the city that strikes your imagination is the Central Market, which I immediately christened "The Belly of Riga." In the past it was the largest indoor market in Europe. Its pavilions are consecutively connected hangars for dirigibles from the time of WWI. It is a grandiose market the like of which you can't find either in Moscow, or in Petersburg, or in Kyiv. It is a pleasure to wander through it. I managed to come across some things here that are specifically Latvian, including a fantastic peasant round rye loaf called "*lachi*" (that is, "of the bear," "from the bear's lair"). Latvians are masters at mixing flour of different kinds and milling. I was also intrigued by the green hemp oil (dopers need not worry about it) and the gray peas (cooked with bacon). However, in the huge fish pavilion I could not find any fresh catch: no Baltic herring, or the legendary lamprey eel, which is sold either fried or jellied, or even fat herring. I was told not to look for the lamprey eel even in restaurants because months that don't have letter "r" in their names are out of season for them.

I licked my lips and headed for Old Riga – to have a bite to eat and drink beer on tap (it's excellent everywhere, not as it used to be in the past) with garlic croutons or the local Parmesan cheese (which has nothing in common with the one Latvia sends to Russia; this one is almost like the Italian). In a Lido chain restaurant where my friend took me on my first day in Riga, the food turned out to be wholly plentiful, tasty, and relatively inexpensive. That was why from that day on I didn't try to find something better but looked for familiar names. There I tasted a famous desert – "bread soup" (it seems to me that before the Revolution of 1917 it was called Limpopo), a semi-aspic, semi-pudding with the taste of barley malt flour and dark rye bread. The almond marzipans in chocolate also deserve your attention. However, in my opinion, Latvians have never known how to make coffee. The local "brewed" coffee can be drunk only with cream, which is no longer of the right quality. Thank God that nowadays you can order a cup of espresso literally everywhere.

Riga is a big city, the size of Vilnius and Tallinn combined. Here, if you make an effort, you'll be able to find something that can be found only deep in the Russian provinces, for example, a classic Soviet "shot-glass bar" and more than one. I need to point out, however, that there are fewer drunks and tourists in Riga than among its neighbors. There recently they started even selling beer just till 10 P.M. In the majority, Rigans behave very decently, like some kind of victorious "middle class." I observed them for a few days and said to my artist friend: "Do you really hope they'll buy your works? Well. Maybe you're thinking of their children – someday in the future…."

Kishinev, Moldova

From the essay "Kishinev Now"
After all, it's alementary, Dr. Watson

The biggest present to future Moldovans was made by the Roman Emperor Trajan, who, after conquering them, founded Dacia. Two years later, it fell apart, but since those times the ancestors of the Moldovans started to speak one of the languages of the Romance group, which made Kishinev natives relatives to the Romans, Parisians, Madridians, and even the inhabitants of infamous Rio de Janeiro. After achieving their independence, the Moldovans received a rare opportunity to perfect their own version of Latin doing agricultural work in different countries of Europe.

Bumping into billboards and posters that had "Alementary" written everywhere in Kishinev, I was forced to think: "Well, Dr. Watson, figure it out, what stands behind it? I wanted to resolve this problem logically, and guessed right – the answer is food stores; they are the institution for which the Moldovan economy works. Where else can you dispatch these kinds of goods that are not brought up to standards? The wine that isn't too bad, but doesn't have stable characteristics, and everything else is just like that. Maybe the only place for it is Russia. There are some qualified workers, but it's not enough. Moldovans are generally good-natured people, and they are becoming angry because they don't understand what has happened and is happening to them – who is the puppet-master? The intellectuals entertain pro-Romanian feelings (after all, they share the same language and writers), but the common people "vote" with their feet" (as migrant workers in Russia), with their tongue (more and more littering their speech with indigestible Russian words), and "for the Communists" (and where would you find those Communists? Those who usurped power today, although they were nothing else but "day laborers," will not yield to the "pauper Romania" – in the villages they still remember how it used to look seventy-eighty years ago). You can call it a "capitalist stagnation" that bumps up against the backwardness of technology when the active will of the population is weakened by the attachment to wine ingrained in them since childhood. Even today old women in villages scold their grown up daughters living in the cities: "Why do you give your child tap water? Don't you have wine in the house?" Even though the best homemade wines, with a heavy-bodied taste, have traces of residual fermentation. Vodka puts a lost soul on display, but wine like that softly envelops him and puts him into a relaxed state. That is why Moldovan *melos* (folk melodies) – music, singing and dances – are always "with a hop," so people don't fall asleep. It's a kind of "techno-folk." Nowadays a large number of urban youth have "gotten hooked on" beer, which nevertheless is not as intoxicating as immature young wine. The Moldovans have learned to brew pretty decent quality light beer.

One of the ways to get acquainted

The best way to get to know a city is through the people who populate it, but for starters, it's a good idea to lose yourself in it and then find yourself once again. On the third day of my stay I measured the entire city center of Kishinev with my feet in every direction and remained quite satisfied with the "catch" of my impressions. I began with the city garden, with Opekushin's life-size bust of Pushkin on a pillar with the inscription in the Moldovan language: "Ku lira nordike…," that is, "Where, sounding the lyre of the northern desert, I wandered…." The monument was erected back in 1885.[78] The citizens of Kishinev could not collect enough money for a monument like the ones in Moscow or Petersburg, but it became the third city that honored the exiled poet who compared himself to Ovid.[79] The only difference between them was that Pushkin was exiled to the south, and Ovid – to the far north (the Ancient Roman poet was stunned by the sight of frozen rivers, but he was never able to get accustomed to the wine frozen in pitchers, which did not prevent the Danube barbarians from chipping it off and gnawing on it).

Nowadays it is a small but the best manicured park in the city. Even California cedars grow in it, although somewhat reluctantly. At the entrance from the central prospect, Romanians, when they ruled

---

78 Klekh is referring here to the monument to Alexander Pushkin created by the sculptor Alexander Opekushun in Moscow in 1885. The monument stands in the Stefan the Great Central Park in the Avenue of Moldovan Writers where it was relocated in 1958.

79 In 8 CE the Emperor Augustus exiled the great Roman poet Publius Ovidius Naso to the town of Tomis in the Kingdom of Thrace (nowadays Romania), which was located at the northern edge of the civilized world. The great Russian poet Alexander Pushkin was exiled from Petersburg to the southern parts of the Russian Empire in 1820. Pushkin first lived in Odessa and then spent time in Kishinev.

Kishinev, put up a monument to Stefan the Great[80] (just as the park, the four-kilometer prospect now bears his name). In a rare part of the park we find an overgrown avenue with busts of the classics of Romanian and Moldovan literature. It seems that composers and artists were not in competition with them. Writers were held in the highest esteem not only in Russia. By the way, the only one who could not accept the collapse of the Soviet Union and who committed suicide was Pavel Botsu, a kind of Moldovan Fadeev.[81]

Above the park, parallel to the central prospect, lies the Street of August 31, 1989 (when the law of the Moldovan language and conversion to the Latin alphabet was passed). This quiet, platan tree-lined street in High Colonial style, like somewhere in Rangoon, absolutely won my heart. I felt the "modest charm" of the vanished empire and could not find any signs of aggression. You couldn't find a better place for those who were not rankled with ambitions to become first in the metropolis. In some humane way I felt the nature of that nostalgia for living at one's pleasure, which one of the last Secretary Generals of the Communist Party, Leonid Brezhnev, felt – it was the root of his strange love for Kishinev. Stalin noticed him: "What a beautiful Moldovan!" and pulled him to Moscow from which there was no way back, except for a visit – in one of the alleyways his toadies built a two-storied residence with an elevator for him.

In other parts of the city I came across a modest villa hidden by a tall fence, the house of Maria Bieshu, the opera singer who won the competition for the "best Cio-Cio-San[82] in the world" as

---

80 Stefan III of Moldova was the Romanian ruler of Moldova between 1457 and 1504.

81 Pavel Botsu was a Soviet Moldovan writer, the Head of the Moldovan Union of Soviet Writers, one of the main proponents of Socialist Realism in Moldova. He committed suicide in 1987. Alexander Fadeev was the most prominent Socialist Realist writer in Stalin's Soviet Russia. In 1939 Fadeev became the General Secretary of the Writers' Union and participated in persecution of those writers who disagreed with Party directives. In the early 1950s Fadeev became disappointed with his own writings and committed suicide in 1956.

82 The main character in Puccini's opera *Madama Butterfly*.

local patriots call her. It must be said that Moldovans take pride in all their famous fellow countrymen – from the modernist sculptor Brancusi and a "Dada" poet Tristan Tsara to heroes of the Russian revolutionary Civil War Mikhail Frunze and Sergei Lazo, and the greatest submariner of all times, Alexander Marinesco, who was decommissioned from his submarine for drinking. Across the road from the villa there was a ruined mansion with columns, but without a roof and windows. A stone's throw from there was a water tower built by Alexander Bernardazzi, who loved historical stylization and filled both Kishinev and Odessa with them. He and Alexei Shchusev, another native of Kishinev, are the main architectural luminaries of this city. The first one decorated it on the border between the 19th and 20th centuries, the second planned it after World War II. The water tower has an observation platform, and one of its levels is set aside as a tiny city museum of Kishinev. In the opposite direction I could see the conservatory and the American Embassy with bored soldiers in pea jackets with fur collars (apparently someone forgot to order them to change uniforms).

...I had to walk through the entire central prospect in idle attempts to find a phone card... and only at the very end of the street I came upon a Moldtelecom store that sold them... This end of the street bumped into an equestrian statue, a big Hajduk (a highwayman in Southeastern and Eastern Europe) and the red brigade commander Kotovsky, who nowadays guarded casinos and banks, which he could no longer rob.[83] Life once again made the "knight's L-shaped move" on the chessboard.

I followed life's example when I wandered onto "Kishinev's Belly" – the gigantic central market that stretched along the main street of the city. In it I was lucky to buy tender sheep-milk feta cheese and golden finely ground corn flour so that I could return to Moscow as a genuine *mamalyga* eater.

---

83 Grigory Kotovsky became famous for being the Commander of the First Red Cavalry Army during the post-revolutionary Russian Civil War 1918-1921. Before the revolution he was a gangster and bank robber.

The traveler is in panic

But I did not have time to say anything substantive! Not about the parliament building that looks like a Tsunami wave; not about the gilded cliff of the President Office, standing directly across from it and rising like a forefinger as a gesture of admonition for the deputies of parliament to remember who they are. Not about the golden *kvas* made out of mill offal, used for the brilliant summer soups *zama* (a traditional Romanian/Moldovan green bean and chicken soup) and *ciorba* (a sour Romanian/Moldovan meat and vegetable soup). Not about an underground night club called the "Black Elephant" and its antithesis the "Aero-café" in a glass tube above the city, which is stylized to resemble a dirigible salon with models of flying machines hanging over the tables. Not about how I was offered a bottle of the cheapest Georgian Saperavi wine for $40 on the empty terrace of a restaurant in the Ryshkanovka district of Kishinev. Apparently someone was laundering money there because in a restaurant on the other side of the street a bottle of the Moldovan premium Cabernet cost ten times less. Three young prostitutes sat at a table nearby. One of them shouted into her cell phone: "Christ, *blin* [eff it], is Risen!"[84]

Kyiv, Ukraine

From an essay about Kreshchatik, "The Main Street of Ukraine"

By his appearance our taxi cab driver looked ridiculously like Stierlitz in disguise ready to meet Borman.[85] But his temperament was very much Neapolitan. He was definitely missing an extra pair of hands because the entire forty-kilometer stretch from the international airport to the

---

84 "Christ is Risen!" is the typical Russian and Ukrainian greeting given during Easter.

85 Klekh is referring to a cult-classic TV series about WWII called "Seventeen Moments of Spring," in which Shtirlitz is a high-placed Russian spy operating in Nazi Germany.

city, he constantly let the steering wheel of his second-hand Volvo go, trying to express with his fingers and in person whatever he was so impatient to convey to us. In particular: how he drives Germans and Turks to their Ukrainian brides, and Donbas "brothers"[86] – to people's Deputies; how he earns money by doing his taxi driving for his son's education to make a diplomat out of him; where you can buy real Kyiv torte – only at the confection factory store!; and also where you could have an inexpensive and satisfying dinner on Kreshschatyk – only in the bistro "Zdorovenki Buly" (Howdy) on the corner of Luteransky (Lutheran) Street! He folded his fingers, indicating that only six first courses would be ten times more expensive at a restaurant and be twice as bad as at home. With his fingers on the steering wheel, he showed me where to go to pick up a tray, and at the same time he diverted his attention and commented, like an inveterate comedian, on every quite trivial occurrence on the street. The photographer and I had immediately "got it" that we were in Ukraine, that it is south where the mixture of self-interest and open-heartedness hits you on the spot, and you don't have to ask anyone about anything – they'll tell you themselves. In the end we wrote down Vasily's – that was the cab driver's name – cell phone number so he could drive us back to the airport at the beginning of next week, making our parting with the Ukrainian capital more pleasant.

The Belly of Kyiv

While the Maidan is the heart of Khreshchatyk, Bessarabsky Square, with the major Kyiv market, is its belly. They say that former Ukrainians in the New World grieve over the *brynza* farmer's cheese "like they have at the Bessarabsky" and other exclusive Ukrainian foods like over nothing else. At the Bessarabsky Market all these foods are of the highest quality, which is proven by their prices. Generally speaking, that year the prices at Ukrainian markets outstripped those of Moscow by 30% - 50% – and it was in Ukraine

---

86 Ukrainian mafia.

where the earth buzzes with fertility and where everything grows, Kyivans could not believe their eyes. But the Bessarabsky Market was a kind of a champion in this respect – a kilogram of homemade ring sausage cost $20 this summer. I ran into this price in Kyiv ridiculously often. It was the price for a taxi from Boryspil Airport to Kyiv (if you are good at haggling, you can cut it in half); for an umbrella on a rainy day bought in the underground passage under Khreshchatyk; for an English-Ukrainian Kyiv guide book (the best one even by today's standards, published in 2001 by the Lviv Publisher "The Center of Europe"). The logic behind it was: they can't give more than that, but we have to ask the maximum, and 100 hryvnas are just that.

Under the roof of the Bessarabka (as it's called by the locals) almost half the space is occupied by flowers and beautiful bouquets of flowers that look like festive cakes – the representatives of various firms (for whom the price of the bouquets does not matter) come to pick them up. There was a lot of red and black contraband caviar – rumor had it that it came from the Sea of Azov. Only a small corner was left for the meat and dairy products, because remodeling was going on in another part of the building. The photographer Alexander and I managed to take a look at the market from above. The guards took us to the director of the market, and he, slightly surprised, kindly agreed to accompany us to the gallery where the administrative offices were located. He made the impression on us of a "person in his place," who knew and loved his business and position, who valued his social status in the city and felt deeply satisfied with it. Everything I knew about the market was known to him: that the building of the Bessarabsky Market was designed in the Art Nouveau style by the Warsaw architect Henryk Gay on the money of the sugar producer Lazar Brodsky and built in 1912 by the Kyivan engineer Bobrusov, who crammed the building with inventive steel construction (he was one of the many who exhibited so-called Russian "white" envy of their French colleague Eiffel – similarly, the colossal indoor market in Riga was constructed in 1920 from the disassembled structures of dirigible hangars). From the gallery windows the market looked like a work of applied art. The director proudly said that the height from the floor to the ceiling in the center of the market was 40 meters. I asked him who were the customers – new Ukrainians? He dodged the answer by saying that people are ready to pay for quality, and this market was never cheap. But it's not true. If you raised your head you would see two reliefs on the front wall – the figures of villagers: a peasant bringing his goods to the city on his oxcart and a milkmaid with a dozen pitchers on a pole, like a crossbeam. Each pitcher held about four-tenths of a liter of milk, weighing about a pound. The customer would drink the cool milk right in the street and, after paying her, returned it back most likely to the barefoot peasant woman. On the side of the Bessarabsky, across the street from it, we met its present day sisters from the villages – right on the sidewalk of Khreshchatyk they spread their vegetables and fruit because their day's earnings would not be enough to pay for a place in the market. Not very far from them sat a man with a cardboard sign "Crayfish" written by hand on it. I asked him where were the crayfish and how much? He said that the price was $12 per kilogram and they were in the trunk of the car over there – in shade of a tree – we can go there. The sun was really hot by then.

Across from the Bessarabsky, on a Sunday morning we had a curious meeting. A nice looking Ukrainian woman (somehow you could see right away that she was Ukrainian) was getting in her foreign car with a breathtaking fruit torte in the shape of a heart in her hands and, to our surprise, engaged us in conversation and posed with her product with the market in the background. She turned out to be no more, no less than chef of the trade center of the Hotel Palace-Royale. Her name was Tatiana; she was going to wish "Happy Birthday" to a Ukrainian TV star; she was born in the Transcarpathian region; she was being driven by her son Dima – an athletic-looking and well-educated guy who had two law degrees at 23 years of age – one from Kyiv and another from Pisa University.

"Oi, you're from *Around the World!*[87] It was my parents' favorite magazine. I remember it from my childhood. Why don't you come to our reception at the Palace-Royale tomorrow!"

Alas, it was the day we had tickets for our return flight to Moscow.

She was a real "southern" woman – lively, blushing and open. She had used Quantro orange peel liqueur for her confectionary masterpiece. I asked her: "Why not Grand Marnier on wild oranges?"

After that we discussed the relative advantages of this or that product sold in fresh and frozen form, exchanged telephone numbers, and parted, mutually enchanted with each other, like Chichikov and Manilov[88] – feeling like: life was good.

When you find yourself on the Maidan, it's worth talking about underground Kyiv. Perhaps, I'm mistaken, but it seems to me that some very archaic layers of the Ukrainian mentality are revealed in the enthusiasm with which Kyivans approach the assimilation of the underground space. It is something that stretches from treasure hunting in Scythian burial mounds and the caves of the Kyivan Monastery of the Caves. Soon after the opening of the Kyiv subway and the construction of the first Ukrainian underground street crossing under European Square, a forked underground street crossing was built under Khreshchatyk, with shops and entrances to the metro, the famous "Tube." Here in the early 1970s the "glass window" shops opened. It was a place where at night you could drink coffee and have a bite to eat as if you weren't in boring Soviet Kyiv, but in some kind of New York City where nightlife was teeming. By the way, even nowadays the "Tube" has tiny establishments that offer quite decent *varenyky* and *draniki*.

---

87 A popular Russian magazine, an equivalent of *National Geographic*.

88 Characters from Nikolai Gogol's novel *Dead Souls*. An adventurist Chichikov comes to the small landowner Manilov to buy names of dead or missing peasants (then called "souls") that still exist in the census books. He needs them to acquire free land from the government on which he planned to settle the non-existent peasants. In Manilov Gogol satirizes the sentimental liberal. Manilov and Chichikov conduct their deal in the most saccharine of tones,

Curiously enough, one more underground trade center Metrograd was built at the other end of Khreshchatyk Street, but in the new century, although it comes off as a "lightweight" against The Globus under the Maidan – it's cramped, the ceilings are low as in the crowded "Tube." Thus The Globus is still the unquestionable favorite of underground Kyiv, and for that reason it's loved by Kyivans who like to stroll here among the expensive boutiques, fountains, and cafes, going from one level to another and hurrying to the still more spacious and stylish The Globus-2 on the opposite side of Khreshchatyk Street. This new Globus has Western-style escalators and glass elevators; it's easy to breathe there because an airplane size propeller fan spins under the cupola itself, and on the bottom they brew wonderful coffee, and there are tables where you can smoke.

If you extract their history from the pre-revolutionary buildings at the end of Khreshchatyk Street, what will you get? The Kozatska Vtikha Tavern (The Cossack's Delight) located deep in an inner courtyard with scents wafting from the kitchen (my restaurateur friend advised me on such occasions to leave immediately – in good restaurants the scent should come from the food, not from the kitchen). Next I searched for the Old Kyiv *varenyky* café, of which I had heard so much from the former Kyivans who feel nostalgic about old times, and I easily found an establishment with such a name. In the middle of the day it was empty, not counting a bored man from the Caucasus Mountains sitting at a table, who turned out to be both the barkeeper and waiter. There were no *varenyky*, and he said the following about his borsht: "What do you want out of borsht, red borsht is borsht even in Africa!" His two answers were enough for me to turn around and leave, and for him – to plop on his chair once again.

Oh, if only this borsht could be truly red, sweet and sour, scorching hot, and with everything it should have in it! Alas, not even once could I have borsht like that in Kyiv – even in establishments with a decent reputation. Why has Ukrainian borsht been discolored to brown? Why everywhere do they call the crude replica without any bone Chicken Kyiv? Why is the steamed crayfish sold by a street vendor at the Konotop railroad platform tastier than those prepared in a Kyivan restaurant? Why in nine out of ten cases can't a Kyivan chef prepare a succulent pork chop? Is it because they don't think you'll come back a second time? The waiters are still sluggish, but already polite, and the chefs are enough to make the saints blush – at best they're interns from a vocational school. I could use an authentic culinary guide for Kyiv, but where can you find one?

Wishing to extract some use of my accidental acquaintance, I asked Tatiana from The Palace Royal Hotel about one of the Khreshchatyk restaurants I wanted to visit before leaving. Her answer was very eloquent: "If I don't know about it, it can't be good!"

Farewell, green city...

It seems the song was sung somewhat differently, and it was about a totally different city, but also a southern one. The business trip had been, generally speaking, a success. The last day the photographer and I spent taking in some fresh air – on the green hill of Poskotina or Honcharka, a fifteen-minute walk from Khreshchatyk. In a store we knew from our previous visit, we bought a few bottles of Shabo white wine,[89] a fresh baguette, and the last piece of Roquefort cheese (with "Rochefort" on the wrapper!), lay down on the grass, and watched the clouds over the Dnipro River basin.

It's a sacred place, and only those who grew up in Kyiv and their friends know about it. The white-bearded patriarch of Ukrainian science fiction[90] maintained that it was a place where a UFO fell –

---

89   The Tatar village of Shabo was established around 1500 and was called Acha-abag ("the lower vineyards"). It emptied after it was occupied by Russians but repopulated by Alexander I in 1822 when Swiss winemakers were brought in to cultivate the vineyards of Shabo. Their descendants continue their business today, and the Shabo wines are appreciated for their qualities.

90   Klekh is referring to Oles Berdnik (1926-2003), a major Ukrainian science fiction writer and the author of almost 30 books. He was one of the founders of a civic rights movement in Ukraine during Soviet times.

and you know who was born out of them. The hill is safe for now: the earth will suck tractors in, your hands will wither away there, etc. However, below and from the sides, it's already surrounded by the elite's new constructions.

It wasn't our hill. We just lay on it – and flew away, let them settle the score by themselves.

Contents

Acknowledgements 7

Introduction 9

Part I: The Philosophy of the Kitchen 19

    The Origin of the Kitchen 20

    The Professor of Sour Cabbage Soup,
    or Homage to William Pokhlebkin 25

    In Defense of Sumptuous Eating 33

    The Sons of Ursa Major 35

    Tell Me What You Eat… 37

    We Do Not Eat It! 39

Part II: Cultural Dictionary of Eastern Slavic Food 43

    Salo (Pig Lard) 45

    The Blin 47

    Kielbasa as a Political Measure 49

    Vodka as Pure Alcohol 51

    The Metaphysics of a Hangover 52

    Soup Therapy 54

    The Invention of Cheese 56

    Hangover Cookery 58

    A Holiday from Nothing, or Polish Bigos 66

The White Gold of Ukraine	70
Syr Dariya District Pilaf	73
Beef Liver Pate and Sardines in Tomato Sauce	75
Wine and Coffee	77

Part III: Seasonal Culinary Art … 45

A Stitch in Time Saves Nine, or It's Really Helpful to Have a Spoon for Dinner	80
The Modest Beauty of the Lenten Table	81
Kholodets (cold jellied meat) is not studen (cold gelatin meat)	83
Pelmeni (meat ravioli) are not Varenyky (cottage cheese or cherry dumplings)	84
Kasha, Porridges, and Gruels	88
Sweets and Whims	90
The Desire for Soup	92
The Formula for Borsht	94
Maslenitsa (Shrovetide), Blin!	100
Fresh Water Carp	102
Wild Salmon	104
Kulichi (Easter Cakes) and Dyed Eggs	106
Pies and Pirozhki	109
Cabbage – it is the Head!	113
Smooth Jams and Lazy Preserves	114
Is eggplant really "blue"?	116
The Kitchen of a Hot Summer Day	122
Salads: Advices and Recipes	126

Five More Kinds of Soup ... 129
Polenta, or in another word – It's Mamalyga ... 132
Fried Potatoes, Boiled Potatoes… ... 134
Pickled and Marinated Vegetables ... 137
Home-made Fast Food ... 141

Part IV: Cities and Dishes ... 144

Hamburg and Munich ... 144
Lobster and Others ... 144
The Munich Strategy ... 147
Berlin, Germany ... 150
Lucerne, Switzerland ... 152
Aqaba, Jordan ... 157
Tomso, Norway ... 159
Vilnius, Lithuania ... 160
Is It Easy to Get Lost in Vilnius? ... 160
Riga, Latvia ... 163
Gates and the Belly of Riga ... 163
Kishinev, Moldova ... 165
One of the ways to get acquainted ... 167
The traveler is in panic ... 170
Kyiv, Ukraine ... 170
The Belly of Kyiv ... 171
Farewell, green city… ... 176

To Get Ukraine
by Oleksandr Shyshko

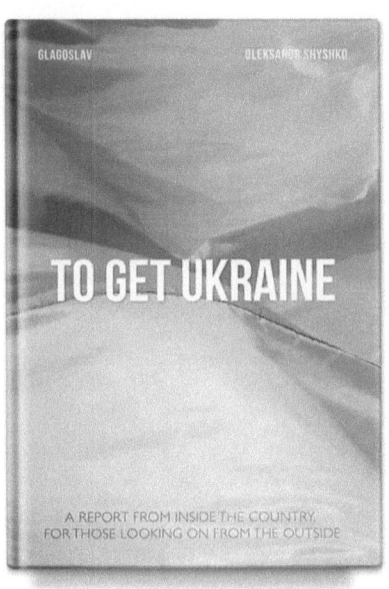

Since Maidan in Kyiv and Russian presence in the Crimea, Ukraine has never been the same. In 2014, the country is deeply divided by the conflict imposed on the Ukrainians. But since nobody actually asked the nation, author Oleksandr Shyshko decided to take matters into his own hands and look for the answer to the ultimate question – who are the Ukrainians and what do they want.

Shyshko spent his time researching the national identity of native Ukrainians, and as he went he stumbled on a discovery that led to yet another question – where is Ukraine going, the so-called Quo vadis? of the Ukrainian people. His findings and critical comments gave birth to this new book that is now for the first time being published in English. To Get Ukraine.

Buy it > www.glagoslav.com

Dear Reader,

Thank you for purchasing this book.

We at Glagoslav Publications are glad to welcome you, and hope that you find our books to be a source of knowledge and inspiration. We want to show the beauty and depth of the Slavic region to everyone looking to expand their horizon and learn something new about different cultures and different people, and we believe that with this book we have managed to do just that.

Now that you've gotten to know us, we want to get to know you. We value communication with our readers and want to hear from you! We offer several options:

– Join our Book Club on Goodreads, Library Thing and Shelfari, and receive special offers and information about our giveaways;

– Share your opinion about our books on Amazon, Barnes & Noble, Waterstones and other bookstores;

– Join us on Facebook and Twitter for updates on our publications and news about our authors;

– Visit our site www.glagoslav.com to check out our Catalogue and subscribe to our Newsletter.

Glagoslav Publications is getting ready to release a new collection and planning some interesting surprises — stay with us to find out more!

Glagoslav Publications
Office 36, 88-90 Hatton Garden
EC1N 8PN London, UK
Tel: + 44 (0) 20 32 86 99 82
Email: contact@glagoslav.com

Glagoslav Publications Catalogue

- The Time of Women by Elena Chizhova
- Sin by Zakhar Prilepin
- Hardly Ever Otherwise by Maria Matios
- Khatyn by Ales Adamovich
- Christened with Crosses by Eduard Kochergin
- The Vital Needs of the Dead by Igor Sakhnovsky
- A Poet and Bin Laden by Hamid Ismailov
- Kobzar by Taras Shevchenko
- White Shanghai by Elvira Baryakina
- The Stone Bridge by Alexander Terekhov
- King Stakh's Wild Hunt by Uladzimir Karatkevich
- Depeche Mode by Serhii Zhadan
- Herstories, An Anthology of New Ukrainian Women Prose Writers
- The Battle of the Sexes Russian Style by Nadezhda Ptushkina
- A Book Without Photographs by Sergey Shargunov
- Sankya by Zakhar Prilepin
- Wolf Messing by Tatiana Lungin
- Good Stalin by Victor Erofeyev
- Solar Plexus by Rustam Ibragimbekov
- Don't Call me a Victim! by Dina Yafasova
- A History of Belarus by Lubov Bazan
- Children's Fashion of the Russian Empire by Alexander Vasiliev
- Boris Yeltsin - The Decade that Shook the World by Boris Minaev
- A Man Of Change - A study of the political life of Boris Yeltsin
- Gnedich by Maria Rybakova
- Marina Tsvetaeva - The Essential Poetry
- Multiple Personalities by Tatyana Shcherbina
- The Investigator by Margarita Khemlin
- Leo Tolstoy – Flight from paradise by Pavel Basinsky
- Moscow in the 1930 by Natalia Gromova
- Prisoner by Anna Nemzer
- Alpine Ballad by Vasil Bykau
- The Complete Correspondence of Hryhory
- The Tale of Aypi by Ak Welsapar
- Selected Poems by Lydia Grigorieva
- The Fantastic Worlds of Yuri Vynnychuk
- The Garden of Divine Songs and Collected Poetry of Hryhory Skovoroda

More coming soon…

www.ingramcontent.com/pod-product-compliance
Lightning Source LLC
Chambersburg PA
CBHW020907080526
44589CB00011B/473